The Primary FRCA Structured Oral Examination Study Guide 1

Second Edition

Lara Wijayasiri and Kate McCombe

Illustrations by Paul Hatton • Foreword by David Bogod

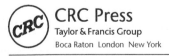

CRC Press
Taylor & Francis Group
Boca Raton London New York

CRC Press is an imprint of the
Taylor & Francis Group, an **informa** business

CRC Press
Taylor & Francis Group
6000 Broken Sound Parkway NW, Suite 300
Boca Raton, FL 33487-2742

© 2017 by Taylor & Francis Group, LLC
CRC Press is an imprint of Taylor & Francis Group, an Informa business

No claim to original U.S. Government works

ISBN-13: 978-1-78523-098-1 (pbk)

Visit the Taylor & Francis Web site at
http://www.taylorandfrancis.com

and the CRC Press Web site at
http://www.crcpress.com

CONTENTS

FOREWORD

Much has happened since I wrote the Foreword to the first edition of this invaluable guide to the Primary FRCA Structured Oral Examination in 2010. Of the three original authors, two have married (each other) and produced a baby girl. One of these two has had to relinquish the authorship of this new edition, since his promotion to the ranks of Primary Examiner unsurprisingly bars him from writing a book on how to pass the Primary exam. The two remaining authors have both moved up the ranks and been appointed as consultants, one with an interest in obstetrics, ethics and law, and the other specialising in vascular anaesthesia and the difficult airway. The first edition, meanwhile, has rapidly become the best-selling textbook on the Primary SOE. If a soap opera was ever to be based around the publication of a guide to passing post-graduate anaesthetic exams – admittedly an unlikely proposition – the story of McCombe and Wijayasiri would surely rival 'EastEnders' for intrigue and plot development.

In this new edition, as well as updating existing topics, the authors have included substantial additions to what was already a very comprehensive book, in line with changes made by the Royal College to the Primary syllabus. The section on 'special patient groups' now includes paediatrics and the elderly, the latter of increasingly personal interest to this writer. The section on physics – often a stumbling block for the Primary candidate – has been extensively revised and now covers those perennial favourites of the examiners, arterial waveforms and vaporisers; as one reads these, there are frequent 'aha!' moments, not least with respect to critical damping, the pumping effect and the influence of altitude on performance. Mindful of the old adage that 'a picture paints a thousand words', the authors have enhanced the number and quality of diagrams and figures, helping to clarify areas such as fetal circulation and the Kreb's cycle.

Some aspects of these books remain, thankfully, unchanged, in particular the resolutely pragmatic approach that McCombe and Wijayasiri take to help readers through the tangled thickets of the Primary. Here are the questions the examiners like to ask, the authors seem to say, and this is how to answer them. It is, perhaps, a tribute to the exam syllabus itself that this approach results in a textbook that is not only very readable but also highly educational.

In short, if you are not lucky enough to be working in the same hospital as the authors, and you cannot approach them for viva practice (or even if you can), then the new edition of this book is an essential companion and a true *vade mecum*. Look it up – a bit of Latin can still impress the examiners!

David Bogod
Consultant Anaesthetist and Ex-Editor-in-Chief of *Anaesthesia*
Nottingham

PREFACE

During our revision for the primary exam we were advised that the best way to ensure success in the structured oral examination (SOE) was to prepare answers to all of the questions in the back of *The Royal College of Anaesthetists Guide to the FRCA Examination, The Primary*. Undoubtedly, this was excellent advice but it proved an enormous task and one we simply did not have time to complete before our own exams. However, once they were over, we began to answer all those questions in the hope that this might help others to prepare for the Primary, or for the basic science component of the Final FRCA. Finally, then, here is the result: the book we wish we'd had.

The Primary FRCA Structured Oral Examination Study Guide provides answers to the questions regularly posed by the examiners. We have not attempted to write the next great anaesthetic textbook, but rather to collate information and deliver it in a relevant and userfriendly layout to make your exam preparation a little easier.

In the SOE itself, each topic will be examined for approximately five minutes. Many of these answers contain much more information than could reasonably be expected of you in that time; however, we have tried to cover several angles of questioning.

We have included the usual chapters on physiology, physics (*Study Guide 1*) and pharmacology (*Study Guide 2*) and, in addition, have written a section on patients who present the anaesthetist with unique problems, 'special patient groups' (*Study Guide 2*). These patients tend to appear in the clinical SOE before some terrible 'critical incident' befalls them. Again, we have included a section addressing the 'critical incidents' beloved of the examiner, with advice as to how to approach them in the SOE (*Study Guide 2*).

There is a unique pharmacology section including information on drugs commonly examined presented in a spider diagram layout. These extremely visual learning aids allowed us to revise the drugs in the necessary detail, and helped us to recall the information even under the acute stress of the exam. We hope you find them just as useful.

We wish you every success in what is undoubtedly a rigorous exam. We believe the key to this success is to practise presenting the knowledge that you already have, logically and concisely. The only way to do this is to practise speaking, even though the possibility of exposing any ignorance is daunting. The more you talk, the more you will cover, and every question is so much easier to answer in the exam if you have already had a dress rehearsal. We hope this book will help you in your preparations.

Good luck!

Lara Wijayasiri
Kate McCombe
December 2015

To Andrew, who makes me believe anything is possible.

Kate McCombe

To Amish, my husband and best friend- thank you for giving me the time to complete this book. And to Maya, my beautiful daughter- thank you for giving me a greater focus in life other than this book.

Lara Wijayasiri

CONTRIBUTORS

Paul Hatton B.Tec
Illustrations

Dr Barbara Lattuca MBBCh MRCP FRCA
Locum Consultant Anaesthetist, St George's NHS Healthcare Trust

Physiology
> Acid-base balance
> Buffers
> Renal blood flow
> Glomerular filtration rate
> Renal handling of glucose, sodium, inulin
> Fluid Compartments
> Osmoregulation
> Baroreceptors
> Immune mechanisms
> Pain pathways

Lt Col Mark Wyldbore MBBS BSc(Hons) FRCA RAMC
Consultant Anaesthetist, Queen Victoria Hospital NHS Foundation Trust

Physiology
> Reflexes

Physics
> General aspects of pressure
> Pressure regulators
> Electrical components
> Defibrillators
> Electrical safety
> Diathermy

ACKNOWLEDGEMENT

Dr Tim Case MBBChir MPhil MA(Cantab)
Our sincerest thanks go to Tim for his eagle eyes and enviable grasp of physics. The book is better for his meticulous reading and attention to detail!

Part 01

PHYSIOLOGY

1. RED BLOOD CELLS AND HAEMOGLOBIN

How are red blood cells (RBCs) produced?	The process of RBC production is called erythropoiesis.

Production of RBCs is controlled by erythropoietin, a hormone produced in the kidneys.

RBCs start as immature cells in the red bone marrow and after about seven days of maturation they are released into the bloodstream. The stages of RBC formation are:

Proerythroblast → Prorubricyte → Rubricyte → Normoblast → Reticulocyte (nucleus ejected by this phase, allowing the centre of the cell to indent giving the cell its biconcave shape – these now squeeze out of the bone marrow and into the circulation) → **Erythroblast**

Hypoxia (e.g. altitude or anaemia) stimulates the kidney to release more erythropoietin, which acts on the red bone marrow where it increases the speed of reticulocyte formation.

How are worn out RBCs removed from the circulation?

RBCs survive for about 120 days. Their cell membranes are exposed to a lot of wear and tear as they squeeze through blood capillaries. Without a nucleus and other organelles, RBCs cannot synthesise new components. Worn out RBCs are removed from the circulation and destroyed by fixed phagocytic macrophages in the spleen and the liver and the breakdown products are recycled.

What happens to the breakdown products of RBCs?

Haemoglobin gets split into its haem and globin components – the globin is broken down into amino acids and the haem gets broken down into iron and biliverdin. The iron combines with the plasma protein transferrin, which transports the iron in the bloodstream. In the muscle, liver and spleen, iron detaches from transferrin and combines with iron-storing proteins – ferritin and haemosiderin. When iron is released from its storage site or absorbed from the gut, it combines with transferrin and gets transported to the bone marrow where it is used for RBC production. Biliverdin gets converted into bilirubin, which enters the circulation and is transported to the liver where it is secreted into the bile.

Why is haemoglobin essential?

Oxygen is relatively insoluble in water and therefore only approximately 1.5% of total oxygen is carried dissolved in the plasma. The remaining 98.5% is bound to haemoglobin. Haemoglobin increases the oxygen-carrying capacity of blood approximately 70-fold.

Describe the molecular structure of haemoglobin.

The haemoglobin molecule is a tetramer composed of four subunits. Each subunit consists of a polypeptide chain (globin) in association with a haem group. A haem group consists of a central charged iron atom held in a ring structure called a porphyrin.

Different forms of haemoglobin exist depending on the structure of these polypeptide chains. In normal adults 98% of all haemoglobin is in the form of HbA1 (2 α chains and 2 β chains). The remaining 2% is in the form of HbA2 (2 α chains and 2 δ chains). Fetal haemoglobin (HbF) is composed of 2 α chains and 2 γ chains. HbF changes to HbA at around six months of life.

What happens to haemoglobin in sickle cell anaemia?

Sickle cell anaemia is an inherited autosomal recessive blood disorder in which there is an abnormal β polypeptide chain due to a genetic mutation in the amino acid sequence where the amino acid valine is replaced by glutamic acid. In the heterozygous state this confers an advantage against malaria as the shortened lifespan of the erythrocyte prevents the blood-borne phase of the mosquito from completing its life cycle. In the homozygous state the abnormal haemoglobin is susceptible to forming solid, non-pliable sickle-like structures when exposed to low PaO_2, causing the erythrocytes to obstruct the microcirculation, leading to painful crises and infarcts.

What happens to haemoglobin in thalassaemia?

Thalassaemia is an inherited autosomal recessive blood disorder in which the genetic defect results in a reduced rate of synthesis of one of the globin chains that make up haemoglobin. This can result in the formation of abnormal haemoglobin molecules, causing anaemia. Thalassaemia can be α or β depending on which globin chain is being underproduced.

Thalassaemia is a quantitative problem where too few globin chains are synthesised, whereas sickle cell anaemia is a qualitative problem with the synthesis of an incorrectly functioning globin chain.

How does oxygen bind to haemoglobin?

Oxygen binds to the ferrous iron (Fe^{2+}) in haemoglobin by forming a reversible bond. There is no oxidative reaction and so the iron atom always remains in the ferrous form. In the condition methaemoglobinaemia, the ferrous iron is oxidised into the ferric (Fe^{3+}) form.

Each molecule of haemoglobin can bind four molecules of oxygen (i.e. one at each ferrous ion within each haem group). There are several factors that influence binding including local oxygen tension, local tissue environment (temperature, CO_2, hydrogen ions and 2,3 DPG) and the allosteric change and cooperative binding behaviour of oxygen to haemoglobin (*see* Chapter 2, 'Oxygen–haemoglobin dissociation curve', for further details).

Can the dissolved fraction of oxygen be dismissed?

Even though dissolved oxygen represents a small fraction of total oxygen-carrying capacity of the blood, it still constitutes an important fraction. Severe anaemia illustrates the point, e.g. for a Jehovah's Witness who has experienced a massive intra-operative haemorrhage and refuses blood transfusion. One therapeutic option would be the use of hyperbaric oxygen therapy; at three atmospheres and using 100% oxygen the dissolved fraction of oxygen would meet total body oxygen requirements.

The dissolved fraction of oxygen is also responsible for triggering the hypoxic respiratory drive. This is of clinical significance in patients with COPD who are chronic CO_2 retainers, because giving them high-flow oxygen to increase their PaO_2 may lead to loss of their hypoxic drive.

In 2008, the British Thoracic Society published guidelines on the use of emergency oxygen in adults. The guidelines recommend that oxygen be administered to patients whose oxygen saturations fall below the target range (94–98% for most acutely ill patients and 88–92% for those at risk of type 2 respiratory failure with raised CO_2 levels in the blood).

2. OXYGEN–HAEMOGLOBIN DISSOCIATION CURVE

Draw the oxygen–haemoglobin dissociation curve (OHDC).

The OHDC is a graph relating the percentage of haemoglobin saturated with oxygen to the partial pressure of oxygen (PO_2).

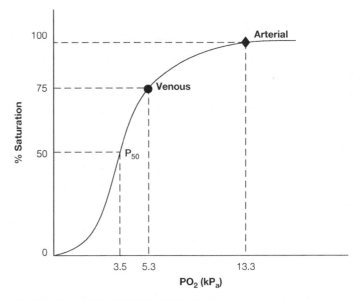

Fig. 2.1 The oxygen–haemoglobin dissociation curve

Normal oxyhaemoglobin dissociation curve

> Arterial PO_2 is 13.3 kP_a with a Hb saturation of 97% (it is not 100% due to venous admixture constituting physiological shunt).
> Venous PO_2 is 5.3 kP_a with a Hb saturation of 75%.
> P_{50} is 3.5 kP_a (this is the PO_2 at which Hb is 50% saturated and it is the conventional point used to compare the oxygen affinity of Hb).

Explain the shape of the OHDC.

The OHDC has a characteristic sigmoid shape due to the binding characteristics of haemoglobin to oxygen:

> **Allosteric modulation**
When oxygen binds to haemoglobin, the two β chains move closer together and change the position of the haem moieties that assume a 'relaxed' or R state. When oxygen dissociates from haemoglobin, the reverse happens and the haem moieties take up a 'tense' or T state.

> **Cooperative binding**
When oxygen binds to haemoglobin the R state is favoured, which has an increased affinity for oxygen and so facilitates the uptake of additional oxygen. The affinity of haemoglobin for the fourth oxygen molecule is, therefore, much greater than that for the first.

What are the major physiological factors that determine the position of the OHDC?

> **Factors that shift the OHDC to the right:** This facilitates the unloading of oxygen into tissues and the P_{50} value is higher than $3.5\,kP_a$:
  • $\downarrow$ pH
  • $\uparrow$ Temperature
  • $\uparrow$ 2,3-Diphosphoglycerate
  • $\uparrow$ $PaCO_2$
  • HbS
  • Anaemia
  • Pregnancy
  • Post-acclimatisation to altitude.

> **Factors that shift the OHDC to the left:** This facilitates the uptake of oxygen from the lungs and the P_{50} value is lower than $3.5\,kP_a$:
  • $\uparrow$ pH
  • $\downarrow$ Temperature
  • $\downarrow$ 2,3-Diphosphoglycerate
  • $\downarrow$ $PaCO_2$
  • HbF
  • Methaemoglobin
  • Carboxyhaemoglobin
  • Stored blood.

What is the Bohr effect?

This describes the right shift in the OHDC in association with increased $PaCO_2$ and hydrogen ion concentration.

What is the double Bohr effect?

This refers to the situation in the placenta where the Bohr effect operates in both the maternal and fetal circulations. The increase in PCO_2 in the maternal intervillous sinuses assists oxygen unloading. The decrease in PCO_2 on the fetal side of the circulation assists oxygen loading. The Bohr effect facilitates the reciprocal exchange of oxygen for carbon dioxide. The double Bohr effect means that the oxygen dissociation curves for maternal HbA and fetal HbF move apart – i.e. right shift (maternal); left shift (fetal).

What is the Haldane effect?

This describes the increased ability of deoxygenated haemoglobin to carry carbon dioxide. Conversely, oxygenated blood has a reduced capacity to carry carbon dioxide. The Haldane effect occurs because deoxygenated haemoglobin is a better proton acceptor than oxyhaemoglobin.

How does the OHDC compare with the myoglobin dissociation curve?

Myoglobin is an oxygen-carrying protein found in skeletal muscles (it gives muscle its dark red appearance).

It consists of a single polypeptide chain associated with a haem moiety.

Unlike haemoglobin, it can only bind one molecule of oxygen and, therefore, its dissociation curve is a rectangular hyperbola.

Myoglobin also has a higher affinity for oxygen than haemoglobin, and so its dissociation curve lies to the left of the OHDC.

Myoglobin takes up oxygen from the circulating haemoglobin and releases it into exercising muscle tissues at very low PO_2, thus providing a source of oxygen during periods of sustained muscle contractions when blood flow to these muscles may be constricted due to blood vessel compression.

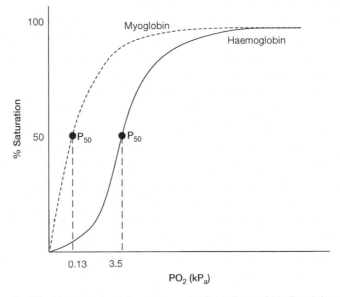

Fig. 2.2 Myoglobin dissociation curve compared to oxyhaemoglobin dissociation curve

3. HYPOXIA

Hypoxia is a core respiratory physiology question and as such examiners will expect a thorough understanding of this topic. Structure your answer.

Define hypoxia and classify the causes.

Hypoxia may be defined either as an inadequate oxygen supply or the inability to utilise oxygen at a cellular level. Causes are divided into four main types:

> **Hypoxic hypoxia** – a $PaO_2 < 12kP_a$
>   - Low FiO_2, e.g. inadvertent hypoxic gas delivery during anaesthesia
>   - Hypoventilation, e.g. opiate induced
>   - Diffusion impairment, e.g. pulmonary oedema, pulmonary fibrosis
>   - Ventilation–perfusion mismatch, e.g. COPD, asthma, LRTI
>   - Shunt, e.g. atelectasis causing intrapulmonary shunt

> **Anaemic hypoxia** – normal PaO_2 but inadequate oxygen-carrying capacity
>   - Low circulating haemoglobin level, e.g. acute and chronic anaemias
>   - Normal circulating haemoglobin level but reduced ability to carry oxygen, e.g. carbon monoxide poisoning

> **Stagnant hypoxia** – normal PaO_2 and oxygen-carrying capacity but reduced tissue and organ perfusion
>   - e.g. cardiogenic shock

> **Histotoxic hypoxia** – normal PaO_2, oxygen-carrying capacity and tissue perfusion but an inability of the tissues to utilise the oxygen at a cellular mitochondrial level
>   - e.g. cyanide poisoning

Draw oxyhaemoglobin dissociation curves showing arterial (♦); and mixed venous (●); points in the four types of hypoxia.

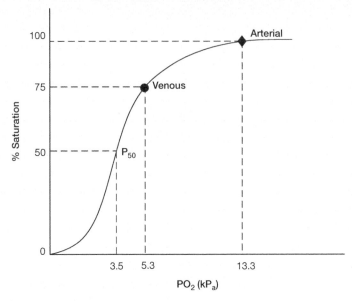

Fig. 3.1   Normal oxyhaemoglobin dissociation curve

> Arterial PaO_2 13.3 kP$_a$.
> Venous $P\bar{v}O_2$ 5.3 kP$_a$.
> P_{50} 3.5 kP$_a$ (partial pressure of oxygen at which haemoglobin is 50% saturated).

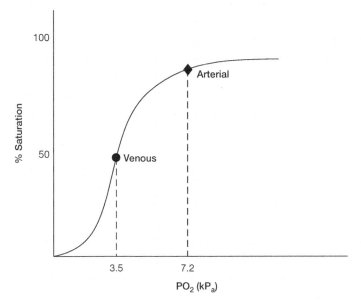

Fig. 3.2   Oxyhaemoglobin dissociation curve in hypoxic hypoxia

> PaO_2 is reduced.
> $P\bar{v}O_2$ is reduced with venous desaturation (<75%).

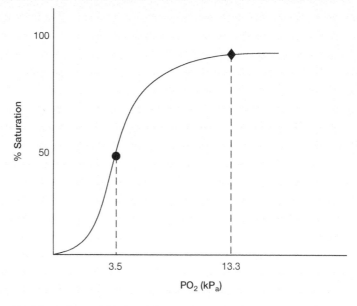

Fig. 3.3 Oxyhaemoglobin dissociation curve in anaemic hypoxia

> PaO_2 remains normal (>13.3 kP$_a$).
> Global oxygen delivery is reduced due to reduced oxygen content.
> Result is increased oxygen extraction and venous desaturation.

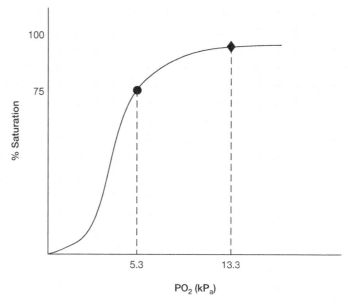

Fig. 3.4 Oxyhaemoglobin dissociation curve in stagnant hypoxia

> PaO_2 is normal.
> $P\bar{v}O_2$ is normal.
> Tissues and organs do not receive the oxygenated blood due to perfusion failure.

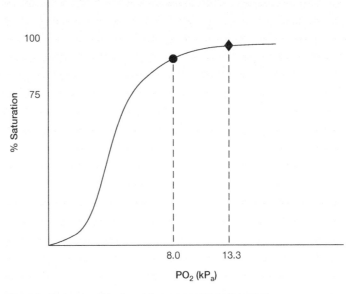

Fig. 3.5 Oxyhaemoglobin dissociation curve in histotoxic hypoxia

> PaO$_2$ is normal.
> Cells are unable to utilise oxygen resulting in high venous saturations.
> Cyanide poisoning will also be associated with a left shift of the oxyhaemoglobin dissociation curve.

What is oxygen content?

Oxygen is carried in the blood in two main ways: combined with haemoglobin and dissolved in the plasma. Oxygen content is calculated by combining the proportion of oxygen bound to haemoglobin with that dissolved.

$$\textbf{Oxygen content = [Bound Oxygen] + [Dissolved Oxygen]}$$
$$\textbf{= [Hb} \cdot \textbf{1.34} \cdot \textbf{SaO}_2\textbf{] + [PaO}_2 \cdot \textbf{0.0225]}$$

Where:
Hb   Haemoglobin g/dL
1.34   Huffner's constant – each gram of haemoglobin combines with 1.34 mL oxygen
SaO$_2$ Arterial oxygen saturation as a percentage, e.g. 96% = 0.96
PaO$_2$ Partial pressure of arterial oxygen
0.0225   mL of oxygen per dL per kP$_a$ of oxygen partial pressure

Thus oxygen content may be calculated for arterial (CaO$_2$) and venous (C$\bar{\text{v}}$O$_2$) blood.

E.g. In arterial blood: Hb 15 g/dL, SaO$_2$ 100% and PaO$_2$ 13.3 kP$_a$

Arterial oxygen content $= [15 \cdot 1.34 \cdot 1.0] + [13.3 \cdot 0.0225]$
$= [20.1] + [0.3]$
$= 20.4$ mL of oxygen per dL

E.g. In venous blood: Hb 15 g/dL, $S\bar{v}O_2$ 75% and $P\bar{v}O_2$ 5.3 kP_a

Venous oxygen content $= [15 \cdot 1.34 \cdot 0.75] + [5.3 \cdot 0.0225]$
$= [15] + [0.2]$
$= 15.2$ mL of oxygen per dL

Note that the difference between arterial and venous oxygen content is just under 5 mL of oxygen per dL. If oxygen content is multiplied by cardiac output, oxygen delivery is obtained.

If circulating volume for a 70 kg man is 80 mL/kg (5600 mL), this equates to an arterial oxygen content of just over 1000 mL and a venous oxygen content of approximately 750 mL.

Discuss arterial and venous oxygen content in the four types of hypoxia.

Hypoxic hypoxia
E.g. Altitude: Hb 15 g/dL, SaO_2 85%, PaO_2 6.5 kP_a, $P\bar{v}O_2$ 3.0 kP_a, $S\bar{v}O_2$ 45%

$CaO_2 = [15 \cdot 1.34 \cdot 0.85] + [6.5 \cdot 0.0225] = 17$ mL O_2/dL
$C\bar{v}O_2 = [15 \cdot 1.34 \cdot 0.45] + [3.0 \cdot 0.0225] = 9$ mL O_2/dL

Note arterial oxygen content is reduced and there is increased oxygen extraction resulting in a lower venous oxygen content.

Anaemic hypoxia
E.g. Haemorrhage: Hb 7 g/dL, SaO_2 100%, PaO_2 13.3 kP_a, $P\bar{v}O_2$ 4.0 kP_a, $S\bar{v}O_2$ 50%

$CaO_2 = [7 \cdot 1.34 \cdot 1.0] + [13.3 \cdot 0.0225] = 10$ mL O_2/dL
$C\bar{v}O_2 = [7 \cdot 1.34 \cdot 0.5] + [4.0 \cdot 00225] = 5$ mL O_2/dL

Significant reduction in arterial oxygen content and hence oxygen delivery to the tissues. There will be a resultant increase in cardiac work in an attempt to maintain oxygen delivery to the tissues.

Stagnant hypoxia
E.g. Cardiogenic shock: Hb 15 g/dL, SaO_2 100%, PaO_2 13.3 kP_a, $P\bar{v}O_2$ 5.3, $S\bar{v}O_2$ 75%

$CaO_2 = [15 \cdot 1.34 \cdot 1.0] + [13.3 \cdot 0.0225] = 20$ mL O_2/dL
$C\bar{v}O_2 = [15 \cdot 1.34 \cdot 0.75] + [5.3 \cdot 0.0225] = 15$ mL O_2/dL

Note arterial oxygen content is normal. However, circulatory dysfunction results in inadequate oxygen delivery to organs and venous saturations may even be increased.

Histotoxic hypoxia
E.g. Cyanide poisoning: Hb 15 g/dL, SaO_2 100%, PaO_2 13.3 kP_a, $P\bar{v}O_2$ 8.0 kP_a, $S\bar{v}O_2$ 90%

$CaO_2 = [15 \cdot 1.34 \cdot 1.0] + [13.3 \cdot 0.0225] = 20$ mL O_2/dL
$C\bar{v}O_2 = [15 \cdot 1.34 \cdot 0.9] + [8.0 \cdot 0.0225] = 18$ mL O_2/dL

Arterial oxygen content is normal. However, at a cellular level there is an inability to utilise oxygen, resulting in high venous oxygen content. This picture may also be seen in severe sepsis where despite adequate oxygen delivery cellular hypoxia remains with high central venous saturations.

4. OXYGEN TRANSPORT

Oxygen transport is a fundamental respiratory physiology question and examiners will expect complete understanding of the topic.

How is oxygen transported from the lungs to the cells of the tissues?

> Ventilation of the lungs supplies oxygen to the alveolus.
> Diffusion of oxygen across the alveolus to the pulmonary capillaries.
> Oxygen carriage by blood (combined with haemoglobin and dissolved in plasma).
> Diffusion from capillary to mitochondria.

What is the oxygen cascade?

The oxygen cascade describes the sequential reduction in PO_2 from atmosphere to cellular mitochondria.

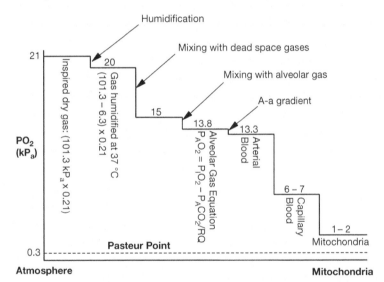

Fig. 4.1 The oxygen cascade

Describe what occurs at each step of the oxygen cascade.

> Oxygen is present in the air at a concentration of 21% (NB. this does not vary with altitude).
> Atmospheric pressure at sea level is 1 atmosphere (or 101 kP_a).
> Inspired PO_2 at sea level is therefore 21 kP_a (atmospheric pressure · % oxygen in air).
> Humidification of inspired air occurs in the upper respiratory tract. The humidity is formed by water vapour, which as a gas exerts a pressure. At 37°C the saturated vapour pressure (SVP) of water in the trachea is 6.3 kP_a. Taking the SVP into account, the PO_2 in the trachea when breathing air is $(101.3–6.3) \times 0.21 = 19.95 kP_a$.
> By the time the oxygen has reached the alveoli the PO_2 has fallen to about 15 kP_a. This is because the PO_2 of the gas in the alveoli (P_AO_2) is a balance between two processes: the removal of oxygen by the pulmonary capillaries and its continual supply by alveolar ventilation (breathing) – thus hypoventilation will result in a lower P_AO_2.
> Blood returning to the heart from the tissues has a low PO_2 (5.3 kP_a) and travels to the lungs via the pulmonary arteries. The pulmonary arteries form pulmonary capillaries, which surround the alveoli. Oxygen diffuses from the high pressure in the alveoli (15 kP_a) to the area of lower pressure of the blood in the pulmonary capillaries (5.3 kP_a).
> After oxygenation blood moves into the pulmonary veins, which return to the left side of the heart to be pumped to the systemic tissues. In a 'perfect lung' the PO_2 of pulmonary venous blood would be equal to the PO_2 in the alveolus. Three factors may cause the PO_2 in the pulmonary veins to be less than the P_AO_2: ventilation/perfusion mismatch, shunt and diffusion impairment. These are the causes of an increased Alveolar–arterial (A–a) gradient.
> Arterial blood with a PaO_2 of 13.3 kP_a passes to the tissues – the capillary PO_2 being in the order of 6–7 kP_a.
> Oxygen then diffuses to the cells in the capillary beds, the mitochondria receiving a PO_2 of 1–5 kP_a depending on the capillary bed.
> An increase in the size of any of the 'steps' in the oxygen cascade may result in hypoxia at the mitochondrial level.

What are the causes of an increased A–a gradient?

Under normal circumstances the A–a gradient is less than 2 kP_a (P_AO_2 15 kP_a and PaO_2 13.3 kP_a) and is caused by small ventilation–perfusion ($\dot{V}/\dot{Q}$) mismatch and shunt present in normal healthy individuals.

However, an increased A–a gradient is present in disease states that result in an increase in $\dot{V}/\dot{Q}$ mismatch/shunt or conditions which impair diffusion.

> **Diffusion impairment**, e.g. pulmonary oedema or pulmonary fibrosis
> **$\dot{V}/\dot{Q}$ mismatch**, e.g. severe hypotension, COPD, LRTI or asthma
> **Shunt:**
> • Intrapulmonary causes, e.g. LRTI or atelectasis
> • Extrapulmonary causes, e.g. right to left cardiac shunt

What are the causes of hypoxia? (see also Chapter 3, 'Hypoxia')

> Low inspired oxygen
> Hypoventilation
> Anaemic hypoxia
> Stagnant hypoxia
> Histotoxic hypoxia
> $\dot{V}/\dot{Q}$ mismatch
> Diffusion impairment
> Shunt

What is the oxygen content in blood?

Oxygen is carried mainly in combination with haemoglobin and also dissolved in plasma.

Each gram of haemoglobin combines with 1.34 mL oxygen (Huffner's constant).

The amount of oxygen dissolved is determined by the partial pressure of oxygen.

$$\text{Oxygen Content} = [\text{Bound Oxygen}] + [\text{Dissolved Oxygen}]$$
$$= [Hb \times 1.34 \times S_aO_2] + [PaO_2 \times 0.0225]$$

Where:

Hb — Haemoglobin (g/dL)

1.34 — Huffner's constant – each gram of haemoglobin combines with 1.34 mL oxygen

SaO$_2$ — Arterial oxygen saturation as a percentage, e.g. 96% = 0.96

PaO$_2$ — Partial pressure of arterial oxygen

0.0225 — mL of oxygen per dL per kP_a of oxygen partial pressure

Thus oxygen content may be calculated for arterial (CaO_2) and mixed venous ($C\bar{v}O_2$) blood.

E.g. In arterial blood: Hb 15 g/dL, SaO_2 100% and PaO_2 13.3 kP_a

Arterial oxygen content $= [15 \times 1.34 \times 1.0] + [13.3 \times 0.0225]$
$= [20.1] + [0.3]$
$= 20.4$ mL of oxygen per dL

E.g. In mixed venous blood: Hb 15 g/dL, 75% and $P\bar{v}O_2$ 5.3 kP_a

Venous oxygen content $= [15 \times 1.34 \times 0.75] + [5.3 \times 0.0225]$
$= [15] + [0.2]$
$= 15.2$ mL of oxygen per dL

Note that the difference between arterial and venous oxygen content is just under 5 mL of oxygen per dL.

If oxygen content is multiplied by cardiac output (heart rate × stroke volume) then oxygen delivery (DO_2) is obtained:

$$DO_2 = CO \cdot CaO_2$$

What methods can be used to increase oxygen content and delivery?

This can be achieved by increasing CaO_2 and or increasing cardiac output (CO).

To increase CaO$_2$:
> Increase circulating haemoglobin concentration (blood transfusion).
> Maintain high oxygen saturations (supplemental oxygen).
> Increase dissolved oxygen by increasing partial pressure of oxygen, e.g. hyperbaric oxygen (achieving a PO_2 of 3 atmospheres supplies sufficient dissolved oxygen to meet oxygen demand).

To increase CO:
> Optimise heart rate and rhythm (rate 60–90 bpm/sinus rhythm).
> Optimise stroke volume (i.e. preload and contractility).
> Maintain perfusion pressure to ensure organ oxygen delivery (i.e. afterload).
> The above can be achieved with the use of fluids and or inotropes.

5. CARBON DIOXIDE TRANSPORT

Normal CO_2 values	Carbon dioxide (CO_2) (MW 44; BP –79 °C; critical temperature 31 °C) is one of the main end products of metabolism. The body contains approximately 120 L of CO_2.

> P_iCO_2 (inspired) $0.03\,kP_a$
> P_ECO_2 (expired) $4\,kP_a$
> P_aCO_2 (arterial) $5.3\,kP_a$
> P_ACO_2 (alveolar) $5.3\,kP_a$ [CO_2 content 21.9 mmol/L]
> P_VCO_2 (venous) $6.1\,kP_a$ [CO_2 content 23.7 mmol/L]

How is CO_2 transported from the cells to the lungs?	Under resting conditions CO_2 production in the body is approximately 200 mL/min. The CO_2 formed in the cells diffuses through the interstitial space to enter the venous circulation.

CO_2 is transported in the blood in three forms:

> **5% dissolved** (CO_2 is 20 times more soluble in blood than O_2)
> **5% carbamino compounds** (combined with NH_2 groups on haemoglobin)
> **90% bicarbonate** (mainly in plasma).

$$CO_2 + H_2O \overset{CA}{\rightleftharpoons} H_2CO_3 \rightleftharpoons H^+ + HCO_3^-$$

Describe the events that take place between the tissue cells and RBCs.	> Reaction between CO_2 and H_2O is slow in the plasma but fast (×1000 faster) within the red blood cell (RBC) due to the intracellular presence of the enzyme carbonic anhydrase (CA).

> HCO_3^- formed in the above reaction diffuses out of the RBC. However, the accompanying H^+ ion cannot follow due to the relative impermeability of the red cell membrane to such cations. In order to maintain electrical neutrality, Cl^- ions diffuse into the red cell from the plasma, the '*chloride shift*'.
> Haldane effect describes how CO_2 transport is affected by the state of oxygenation of Hb. This is because deoxyhaemoglobin is better than oxyhaemoglobin in:
>   • Combining with CO_2 to form carbamino compounds (in turn assisting the blood to load more CO_2 from tissues for removal at the lungs)
>   • Combining with H^+ ions (in turn assisting the blood to load more CO_2 from the tissues)
> As CO_2 leaves the tissue cells and enters the RBCs, it causes more O_2 to dissociate from Hb (Bohr shift) and thus more CO_2 combines with Hb and more HCO_3^+ is produced.

Draw the events that take place between tissue cells and RBCs.

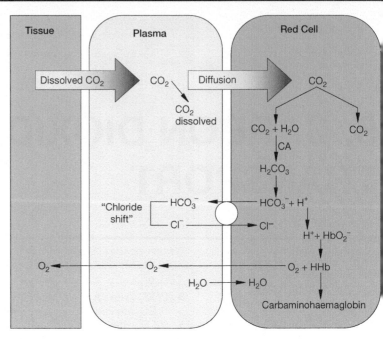

Fig. 5.1   Schematic representation of CO_2 transport between tissue cells and RBCs

Compare the CO_2 dissociation curve with HbO_2 dissociation curve.

CO_2 dissociation curve is influenced by the state of oxygenation of the Hb (Haldane effect) where oxyhaemoglobin carries less CO_2 than deoxyhaemoglobin for the same PCO_2.

CO_2 dissociation curve is more linear than the oxyhaemoglobin dissociation curve which is sigmoid in shape.

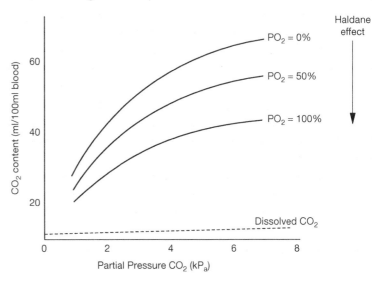

Fig. 5.2 CO_2 dissociation curve at different O_2 saturations

Draw the physiological dissociation curve for CO$_2$.

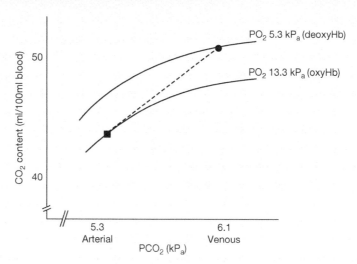

Fig. 5.3 CO$_2$ dissociation curve

6. ALVEOLAR GAS EQUATION

The alveolar gas equation allows you to calculate the alveolar partial pressure of oxygen for a given inspired pressure of oxygen and a given alveolar pressure of carbon dioxide.

The examiners may ask about the alveolar gas equation in various guises ranging from a direct question such as, 'how can the partial pressure of oxygen in alveolar gas be measured?' to 'what effect would sudden decompression of a commercial aircraft at an altitude of 35 000 ft have on alveolar oxygen pressure?'

Irrespective of the format of the question it is vital to understand the key role that the alveolar gas equation plays in understanding the causes of hypoxia and ultimately understanding the alveolar–arterial oxygen difference (A–a gradient).

Write the alveolar gas equation.

$$P_AO_2 = P_iO_2 - \frac{P_ACO_2}{R}$$

Where:

P_AO_2	Alveolar partial pressure of oxygen
P_iO_2	Inspired pressure of oxygen
P_ACO_2	Alveolar partial pressure of carbon dioxide (approximates with $PaCO_2$ due to rapid diffusion of CO_2)
R	Respiratory Quotient = CO_2 production / O_2 consumption (N = 0.8).

Explain how P_iO_2 is calculated.

Inspired O_2 is different from atmospheric O_2 because it is warmed and contains added water vapour. Fractional inspired O_2 does not vary with altitude. However, barometric pressure falls with increasing altitude; halving every 18 000 ft. Partial pressure of water vapour remains constant at 47 mmHg (6.3 kP$_a$). Thus:

$$P_iO_2 = F_iO_2 \cdot (P_{atm} - P_{H_2O})$$

E.g. At sea level (barometric pressure 760 mmHg or 101 kP$_a$)

$$P_iO_2 = 0.21 \cdot (101 - 6.3) = 19.9 \, kP_a$$

E.g. At an altitude of 63 000 ft (barometric pressure 47 mmHg or 6.3 kP$_a$)

$$P_iO_2 = 0.21 \cdot (6.3 - 6.3) = 0$$

At 63 000 ft barometric pressure is equal to the partial pressure of water and therefore a person's blood would boil (as saturated vapour pressure of water would be equal to barometric pressure).

What factors affect the respiratory quotient (RQ)?

The metabolic substrates used are the main determinants of the RQ.

> Carbohydrate RQ 1.0
> Protein RQ 0.8–0.9
> Fat RQ 0.7

Why may P_AO_2 and PaO_2 differ?

If P_iO_2 is held constant and $PaCO_2$ increases, P_AO_2 and PaO_2 will always decrease. Since P_AO_2 is a calculation based on known (or assumed) factors, its change is predictable. PaO_2, by contrast, is a measurement whose theoretical maximum value is defined by P_AO_2 but whose lower limit is determined by ventilation–perfusion ($\dot{V}/\dot{Q}$) imbalance, pulmonary diffusing capacity and oxygen content of blood entering the pulmonary artery (mixed venous blood). In particular, the greater the imbalance of ventilation–perfusion ratios, the more PaO_2 tends to differ from the calculated P_AO_2. (The difference between P_AO_2 and PaO_2 is commonly referred to as the 'A–a gradient'. However, 'gradient' is a misnomer since the difference is not due to any diffusion gradient, but instead to $\dot{V}/\dot{Q}$ imbalance and/or right to left shunting of blood past ventilating alveoli. Hence 'A–a O_2 difference' is the more appropriate term.)

What is the normal A–a gradient?

The A–a gradient varies with age and FiO_2. Up to middle age, breathing ambient air, the normal A–a gradient is approximately $1.3\,kP_a$ (10 mmHg). Breathing an FiO_2 of 1.0 the normal A–a gradient ranges up to about $10\,kP_a$. If the A–a gradient is increased above normal, there is a defect of gas transfer within the lungs; this defect is almost always due to $\dot{V}/\dot{Q}$ imbalance.

What are the common causes of an increased A–a gradient?

There are three common causes:

> **Ventilation–perfusion ($\dot{V}/\dot{Q}$) mismatching** – blood flowing through high $\dot{V}/\dot{Q}$ areas with a higher PO_2 cannot compensate for the blood flowing through low $\dot{V}/\dot{Q}$ areas because of the shape of the oxyhaemoglobin dissociation curve and because more of the pulmonary blood usually flows through low $\dot{V}/\dot{Q}$ areas.
> **Diffusion impairment** – may occur in conditions such as pulmonary fibrosis and pulmonary oedema. It may also occur if P_iO_2 is low (e.g. high altitude) or if lung capillary transit time is greatly reduced from its normal 0.75 seconds (e.g. exercise).
> **Anatomical shunt** – an extreme form of $\dot{V}/\dot{Q}$ mismatch where deoxygenated blood enters the systemic circulation.

Draw a curve to demonstrate how changes in minute ventilation affect the partial pressures of alveolar oxygen and alveolar carbon dioxide.

As minute ventilation increases, $PaCO_2$ and hence P_ACO_2 decreases ($PaCO_2$ approximates P_ACO_2 due to the rapid diffusion of CO_2). This results in a reciprocal increase in P_AO_2.

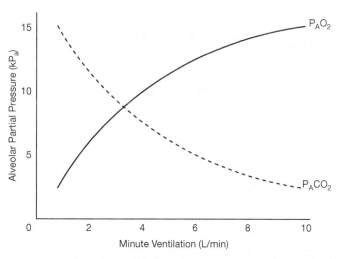

Fig. 6.1 The effect of changes in minute ventilation on P_AO_2 and P_ACO_2

7. VENTILATION–PERFUSION ($\dot{V}/\dot{Q}$) MISMATCH AND SHUNT

What is the ventilation–perfusion ratio?

The ventilation–perfusion ($\dot{V}/\dot{Q}$) ratio is the ratio between the amount of air getting to the alveoli (the alveolar ventilation, V_A, in L/min) and the amount of blood entering the lungs (the cardiac output, Q, in L/min).

Calculating the $\dot{V}/\dot{Q}$ ratio is easy:

$\dot{V}/\dot{Q}$ ratio = alveolar ventilation/cardiac output

If alveolar ventilation is 4L/min and cardiac output is 5L/min then:

$$\dot{V}/\dot{Q} \text{ ratio} = 4/5 = 0.8$$

However, this ratio of 0.8 is only an overall ratio as in reality ventilation and perfusion vary across the lung resulting in a range of $\dot{V}/\dot{Q}$ ratios.

In areas of dead space (i.e. areas that are ventilated but not perfused, e.g. pulmonary embolus) the $\dot{V}/\dot{Q}$ ratio is infinity (because mathematically dividing by zero produces the answer of infinity).

$$\text{Dead space } \dot{V}/\dot{Q} \text{ ratio} = \text{infinity}$$

In areas of shunt (i.e. areas that are perfused but not ventilated, e.g. physiological shunt such as an inhaled foreign body or anatomical shunt such as a right-to-left shunt) the $\dot{V}/\dot{Q}$ ratio is zero (because mathematically dividing zero by any number is always zero).

$$\text{Shunt } \dot{V}/\dot{Q} \text{ ratio} = \text{zero}$$

If ventilation and perfusion are not matched, the consequences for gas exchange are impairment of both O_2 uptake and CO_2 elimination.

How does ventilation vary from the apex to the base of the lung?

> The lungs are suspended within the thoracic cavity and therefore the alveoli are subjected to the effects of gravity.
> In the upright lung intrapleural pressure varies from the top to the base of the lungs. For every centimetre of vertical displacement from the tip of the lung to the base, intrapleural pressure increases by about 0.2 cm H_2O.
> For an average healthy male, the intrapleural pressure at the apex of the lung is about –8 cm H_2O and at the base is about –1.5 cm H_2O. This means that the alveoli at the apex are exposed to a greater distending pressure compared to those at the base.

> Consequently, the alveoli at the lung apex are relatively larger than those at the bases. The apical alveoli are thus on a flatter part of their pressure–volume (i.e. compliance) curve than the basal alveoli, which are on the steep portion of the compliance curve. Therefore, being relatively more compliant, the alveoli at the base fill to a greater extent for a given change in intrapleural pressure during inspiration compared to the alveoli at the apex. Hence, ventilation is preferentially distributed to the basal alveoli.

How does perfusion vary from the apex to the base of the lung?

> The pulmonary circulation is a low-pressure, low-resistance system and is subject to alveolar pressures.
> In an upright, healthy individual at rest, pulmonary blood flow is distributed unevenly through the lung. Similar to the distribution of ventilation, pulmonary blood flow is preferentially directed to the base of the lungs.
> This distribution is dependent on three relative pressures: alveolar pressure (PA), pulmonary arterial pressure (Pa) and pulmonary venous pressure (Pv). On the basis of these pressure relationships, three functional zones are described (West zones).

- Zone 1 (apex): PA > Pa > Pv

Alveolar pressure exceeds vascular pressures resulting in capillary collapse and no blood flow. The alveoli in this zone do not participate in gas exchange and are part of the lung's alveolar dead space. In healthy subjects zone I does not exist because arterial pressures are just sufficient to raise blood to the top of the lung and exceed alveolar pressure. Zone 1 may be present in cases of severe hypotension (e.g. following major haemorrhage) as pulmonary arterial pressure is reduced or if alveolar pressure is raised (e.g. during positive pressure ventilation).

- Zone II (middle): Pa > PA > Pv

Driving pressure for blood flow is now determined by the difference between arterial and alveolar pressures. Alveolar pressure remains constant throughout the lung whereas arterial pressure increases from the apex to the base due to the increase in blood hydrostatic pressure. Therefore, blood flow gradually increases down zone II as the driving pressure (Pa-PA) gradually increases.

- Zone III (base): Pa > Pv > PA

Now both vascular pressures are greater than alveolar pressure and the driving pressure for blood flow is simply pulmonary arterial pressure minus pulmonary venous pressure. The increase in blood flow in zones II and III reflects also the recruitment and distention of pulmonary vessels with increasing intravascular pressures down the lung.

What factors can cause shifts within the West zones?

West zones are physiological boundaries in the lung that are based upon the relationship between the pressure in the alveoli, arteries and veins. The boundaries between these zones can shift due to physiological and pathophysiological changes.

> In healthy subjects, zone I does not exist because arterial pressures are just sufficient to raise blood to the top of the lung and exceed alveolar pressure. Zone 1 may be present in cases of severe hypotension (e.g. following major haemorrhage) as pulmonary arterial pressure is reduced or with a pulmonary embolus as pulmonary artery perfusion will be disrupted.
> Conversely, during exercise pulmonary artery pressure is high eliminating any existing zone I into zone II and moving the boundary between zone III and zone II upward.
> Alveolar pressures are increased during positive pressure ventilation, which can result in substantial areas of lung to fall into zone I.
> Changes in body position alter the orientation of the zones with respect to the anatomic locations in the lung but the same relationship with respect to gravity and vascular pressure remains.

Draw a graph to show how ventilation and perfusion are distributed across the lung.

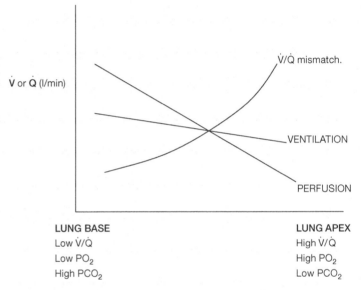

Fig. 7.1 Distribution of ventilation and perfusion across the lung (in a person spontaneously breathing and standing)

Discuss the effects of high and low $\dot{V}/\dot{Q}$ on alveolar O_2 and CO_2 partial pressures.

> The alveolar partial pressure of oxygen and carbon dioxide are determined by the ratio of ventilation to perfusion, which varies across the lung. In the upright position, the gradient for perfusion is greater than that for ventilation.
> At the apex of the lung, $\dot{V}/\dot{Q}$ ratio is highest (about 3.0). Here PaO_2 is highest and $PaCO_2$ is lowest (this explains why organisms that thrive in high O_2 such as TB flourish in the lung apex).
> At the base of the lung, $\dot{V}/\dot{Q}$ ratio is lowest (about 0.6) and now PaO_2 is lowest and $PaCO_2$ is highest.

With a patient in the lateral position, how is ventilation distributed in the following situations: awake patient, anaesthetised patient breathing spontaneously (GA/SV), anaesthetised and ventilated patient (GA/IPPV) and patient with an upper-chest thoracotomy?

	Upper lung (V)	Lower lung (V)
Awake	40%	60%
GA/SV	55%	45%
GA/IPPV	60%	40%
Thoracotomy	70%	30%

Why are the above changes in ventilation distribution seen?

The explanation centres on the effect of anaesthesia on lung volume and hence the change in compliance of different areas of the lung. The lung pressure–volume curve illustrates the regional variation in lung compliance and shows how under anaesthesia the alveoli at the top of the lung (in the upper lung) move to a steeper portion of the compliance curve as their resting volume falls. Conversely, the basal alveoli (in the lower lung) move to a flatter, less compliant part of the curve.

Lung pressure–volume curve

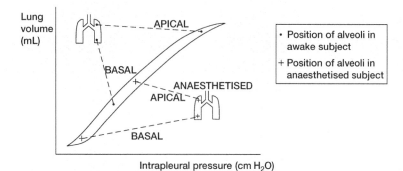

Fig. 7.2   Lung pressure–volume curve illustrating the effect of anaesthesia on lung compliance

Note how under anaesthesia lung volume falls; the alveoli in the upper lung have a reduced volume resulting in increased compliance and hence improved ventilation. The alveoli in the lower lung also undergo volume reduction under anaesthesia. However, the reduction in volume leaves the lower lung alveoli less compliant and, therefore, ventilation is reduced.

What do you understand by the term 'shunt'?

Shunt is an extreme form of $\dot{V}/\dot{Q}$ mismatch, whereby blood enters the arterial system without passing through ventilated areas of the lung. It may be classified into intrapulmonary and extrapulmonary causes.

What are the causes of shunt?

> **Intrapulmonary:**
>   • Physiological: Bronchial arterial blood passing into the pulmonary veins. Coronary venous blood draining into the left ventricle.
>   • Pathological: Lung collapse or consolidation with loss of ventilation.

> **Extrapulmonary:**
>   • Cyanotic congenital heart disease, i.e. right-to-left intracardiac shunting, e.g. Tetralogy of Fallot.

What is the shunt equation?

The shunt equation allows the amount of shunt caused by the addition of venous blood to the arterial circulation to be calculated. It requires the subject to be breathing 100% oxygen. Of fundamental importance is the fact that of all of the causes of hypoxia, shunt cannot be corrected by breathing 100% oxygen because the shunted blood bypasses ventilated alveoli and thus is never exposed to the higher alveolar PO_2. The shunted blood therefore continues to depress the arterial oxygen content.

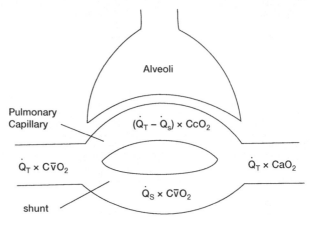

Fig. 7.3 Schematic representation of shunt

$$\frac{\dot{Q}_S}{\dot{Q}_T} = \frac{CcO_2 - CaO_2}{CcO_2 - C\bar{v}O_2}$$

Where:

$\dot{Q}_T$	Total blood flow (measured via cardiac output monitors)
$\dot{Q}_S$	Shunt blood flow
CcO_2	End-capillary oxygen content (estimated from alveolar gas equation)
CaO_2	Arterial oxygen content (ABG then calculate oxygen content)
$C\bar{v}O_2$	Mixed venous oxygen content (mixed venous blood sample from a PAFC then calculate venous oxygen content).

Draw the iso-shunt diagram.

The iso-shunt diagram demonstrates the arterial oxygen tension based on a given inspired oxygen fraction in the presence of various degrees of shunt:

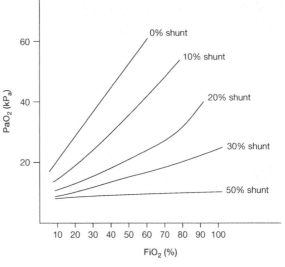

Fig. 7.4 Iso-shunt diagram

8. RESPIRATORY DEAD SPACE

Questions on respiratory dead space are particularly common in the primary FRCA examination. Examiners will expect clear definitions of what constitutes the different types of dead space and how they can be measured.

Define dead space as applied to the respiratory system.

Respiratory dead space is the volume of inspired gas that does not take part in gas exchange. It is divided into anatomical and alveolar dead space.

> **Anatomical dead space:**
>   • Constitutes the conducting airways (Weibel classification – airway generations 1–16: trachea, bronchi, bronchioles and terminal bronchioles)
>   • Includes the mouth, nose and pharynx
>   • Equates to 2 mL/kg

Table 8.1 Factors affecting anatomical dead space

Anatomical dead space increased by:	Anatomical dead space decreased by:
Sitting up	General anaesthesia
Neck extension and Jaw protrusion	Hypoventilation
Increasing age	Intubation
Increasing lung volume	Tracheostomy

> **Alveolar dead space:**
>   • Constitutes alveoli that are ventilated but not perfused and, therefore, no gas exchange occurs
>   • Can be significantly affected by physiological and pathological processes

> **Physiological dead space:**
>   • Represents the combination of anatomical and alveolar dead space

How is anatomical dead space measured?

Fowler's method is used to measure anatomical dead space. It is a technique that uses single-breath nitrogen washout utilising a rapid nitrogen gas analyser.

> A nose clip is placed on the subject, and the subject breathes air in and out through their mouth via a mouthpiece.
> From the end of a normal expiratory breath (i.e. FRC) the subject takes a maximal breath of 100% O_2 to vital capacity.
> Subject then exhales maximally at a slow and constant rate to residual volume.
> During exhalation the expired gas passes through the rapid nitrogen analyser and so nitrogen concentration is measured against volume.
> Four distinct phases are seen in expired nitrogen concentration.

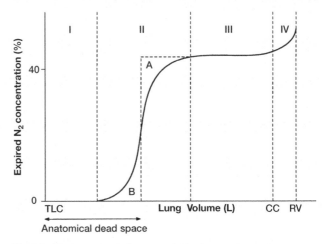

Fig. 8.2 Nitrogen concentration versus lung volume

> **Phase I:** Initial expired gas from the conducting airways containing 100% O_2 and no N_2.
> **Phase II:** Nitrogen concentration increases as alveolar gas begins to mix with anatomical dead space gas.
> **Phase III:** Alveolar plateau phase – exhalation of alveolar gas containing N_2 from the alveoli. Oscillations can be seen in phase 3, which are caused by interference from the heartbeat.
> **Phase IV:** Represents closing capacity. During expiration airways at the lung bases close as the lung approaches residual volume, so phase 4 expired gas comes mainly from the upper lung regions. During normal inspiration the lung bases are preferentially ventilated and therefore the lung apices receive less of the 100% O_2 breath. At closing volume N_2 from the lung apices is expired causing the phase 4 rise in expired N_2 concentration.
> **Anatomical dead space** is found by dividing phase 2 so that areas A and B are equal and measuring from the start of exhalation.

How is physiological dead space measured?

The Bohr equation is used to derive physiological dead space (anatomical + alveolar).

$$\frac{V_{D.PHYS}}{V_T} = \frac{PaCO_2 - P_ECO_2}{PaCO_2}$$

Where:

$V_{D.PHYS}$ Physiological dead space

V_T   Tidal volume – measured with a spirometer

$PaCO_2$ Arterial partial pressure of CO_2 – measured from an arterial blood gas

P_ECO_2   Mixed expired partial pressure of CO_2 – measured from end-tidal CO_2.

Any of the situations previously mentioned that increase anatomical dead space will consequently increase physiological dead space.

Alveolar dead space is increased by most lung diseases (especially pulmonary embolus), general anaesthesia, positive pressure ventilation and positive end expiratory pressure. Under such circumstances $V_{D.PHYS}/V_T$ may approach 70% (normally 35%), which has obvious implications for CO_2 removal.

9. LUNG VOLUMES

Draw a spirometer trace to illustrate the various lung volumes.

Spirometry is the standard method for measuring most relative lung volumes. However, it is incapable of providing information about absolute volumes of air in the lung. Thus a different approach is required to measure residual volume, functional residual capacity and total lung capacity. Two of the most common methods of obtaining information about these volumes are gas dilution tests and body plethysmography.

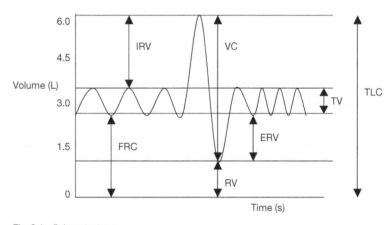

Fig. 9.1 Spirometry trace

All values quoted are approximate for a 70-kg man:

TLC   Total lung capacity (6000 mL)
VC   Vital capacity (4800 mL)
TV   Tidal volume (400–600 mL)
IRV   Inspiratory reserve volume (2500 mL)
ERV   Expiratory reserve volume (1200 mL)
RV   Residual volume (1200–1500 mL)
FRC   Functional residual capacity (3000 mL standing up or 2000 mL supine).

Which lung volumes can be measured with a spirometer?

Any lung volume that incorporates residual volume cannot be measured with simple spirometry (i.e. TLC, RV and FRC), the rest can be measured:

> **Vital capacity** – the maximum volume expired after a maximal inspiration
> **Tidal volume** – normal resting breath volume
> **Inspiratory reserve volume** – volume of air that can be inspired over and above the resting tidal volume
> **Expiratory reserve volume** – volume of air that can be expired from end of normal tidal volume.

How can absolute lung volumes be measured?

The absolute lung volumes are:

> **Residual volume** – volume of air remaining in the lungs after maximal expiration
> **Total lung capacity** – total volume of air in the lungs after maximal inspiration
> **Functional residual capacity** – volume of air remaining in the lungs after a normal expiratory breath

These cannot be measured by simple spirometry, but require the use of more advanced techniques such as **gas dilution** or **body plethysmography**.

Describe how nitrogen washout may be used to measure RV and FRC.

> The fractional lung nitrogen concentration (FLN$_2$) is constant at 79% (i.e. 790 mL per 1000 mL air). The subject rebreathes several times from a bag of known volume containing a nitrogen-free gas. Thus, the nitrogen from the patient's lungs equilibrates with gas in the bag and so the nitrogen concentration will decrease as the volume of distribution has increased.
> In order to measure RV, the rebreathing process is started from the end of a maximal expiration (i.e. from RV).
> In order to measure FRC, the rebreathing process is started from the end of a normal tidal breath (i.e. from FRC).
> The principle behind the nitrogen washout method is that the amount of nitrogen at the start of the determination (nitrogen in the patient's lungs only) is the same amount that ultimately is distributed between the lung and the bag. As the volume of the bag and the fractional concentration of nitrogen in the lungs are known, the fractional concentration of nitrogen in the bag at equilibration is measured, allowing calculation of either RV or FRC.

Thus:

$$VL = \frac{VB \cdot FxN_2}{FLN_2 - FxN_2}$$

Where:
VL   Volume of lung (FRC or RV)
VB   Volume of bag
FxN$_2$ Fractional concentration of N$_2$ in bag
FLN$_2$ Fractional concentration of N$_2$ in the lung

Exactly the same principle is used for the helium wash-in method of determining RV or FRC. Both the nitrogen washout and helium wash-in methods measure only communicating gas. This is a disadvantage compared to the total body plethysmography method, which is able to measure communicating and non-communicating gas (i.e. gas trapped behind closed airways).

Describe how body plethysmography may be used to measure RV and FRC.

> The subject sits inside an airtight chamber equipped to measure pressure, flow or volume changes.
> The subject inhales or exhales to a particular volume (usually FRC), and then a shutter drops across their breathing tube.
> The subject makes respiratory efforts against the closed shutter, causing their chest volume to expand and decompressing the air in their lungs.
> The increase in their chest volume slightly reduces the box volume and thus slightly increases the pressure in the box.
> The most common measurements made using the body plethysmograph are thoracic gas volume and airway resistance.

The following equation is then used:

$$\text{Pressure 1} \cdot \text{Volume 1} = \text{Pressure 2} \cdot (\text{Volume 1} - \text{Volume 2})$$

(It uses Boyle's law – at a constant temperature, within a closed system, pressure is inversely proportional to volume.)

What determines FRC?

FRC is dependent on the balance of the tendency of the lungs to recoil and the thoracic cage to expand.

Under conditions of apnoea, FRC represents the pulmonary oxygen store. If FRC is 2500 mL, breathing 21% O_2 the oxygen store is 500 mL, but this can be increased by preoxygenation (denitrogenation) to 2500 mL. If resting total body O_2 requirement is 250 mL/min, FRC represents a 10 minute O_2 store during apnoea.

> **FRC is increased by:**
> - Standing position
> - COPD
> - Asthma
> - PEEP.

> **FRC is reduced by:**
> - Supine position
> - General anaesthesia
> - Pregnancy
> - Obesity.

What is closing capacity?

The closing capacity is the volume of the lungs at which the small airways begin to collapse and close off. If FRC is less than the closing capacity, areas of the lung will be perfused but not ventilated, resulting in an increase in $\dot{V}/\dot{Q}$ mismatch.

10. LUNG COMPLIANCE

Define lung compliance.

Compliance is the measure of distensibility – the ease at which something can be stretched. Lung compliance (C_L) is defined as the change in lung volume (ΔV) per unit change in transpulmonary pressure (ΔP).

$$C_L = \Delta V/\Delta P$$

> **Specific compliance** is compliance divided by FRC, thereby compensating for differing body sizes.
> **Elastance** is the reciprocal of compliance.

Draw a pressure–volume curve of the lung.

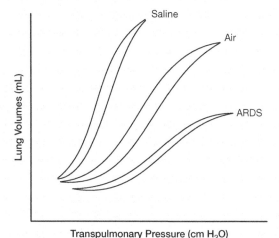

Fig. 10.1 Lung compliance

> Lung compliance is best described using pressure–volume curves of the lungs under static conditions (i.e. when there is no gas flow and the respiratory muscles are relaxed). Under these conditions the transpulmonary pressure reflects in magnitude the elastic recoil pressure of the lungs. The slope of the pressure–volume curve equates to lung compliance. Normal lung compliance is 200 mL/cm H_2O.
> In neonatal respiratory distress syndrome, lung compliance is greatly reduced due to insufficient surfactant.
> Conversely, in hypothetical saline-filled lungs, compliance is greatly increased as the lack of an air–fluid interface means that no surface tension exists.

What do you understand by the term *hysteresis*?

Hysteresis is an important phenomenon seen in P-V curves; it represents 'unrecoverable' energy because the lungs do not act as a perfect elastic system (i.e. a system in which any energy that is put in is immediately returned). At any given lung volume, the pressure required to inflate the lung is greater than that required for deflation.

What is the difference between static and dynamic compliance?

Static compliance is the lung compliance obtained during 'static' conditions when there is no gas flow activity within the lungs. Static compliance monitors only elastic resistance (i.e. the resistance offered by the alveoli being stretched and the interstitium and chest wall being moved). The static compliance curve can be used to select the ideal level of PEEP during mechanical ventilation.

Dynamic compliance is the lung compliance obtained under 'dynamic' conditions when gas flow activity is present during rhythmic breathing. Dynamic compliance monitors both elastic resistance and airway resistance (which depends on gas viscosity and density, length and radius of lumen, gas flow rate and flow pattern).

How can static and dynamic compliance be measured?

Static compliance: This is obtained under 'static' conditions when there is no gas flow (e.g. during an inspiratory pause). The subject breathes into a spirometer to measure lung volumes and an oesophageal pressure probe is used to estimate intrapleural pressures. The volumes and pressures measured are then plotted to produce a pressure–volume curve. The compliance is then calculated from the gradient of the curve (usually measured near FRC). The term 'static' is somewhat misleading because measurements have to be interrupted to allow the subject to breath and therefore the system never truly reaches static conditions (it is, therefore, sometimes called 'quasi-static' compliance).

Dynamic compliance: This is obtained under 'dynamic' conditions when there is gas flow (i.e. during rhythmic breathing). Again the subject breathes into a spirometer to measure lung volumes and an oesophageal probe is used to estimate intrapleural pressures. The term 'dynamic compliance' is also somewhat confusing as the compliance is typically calculated during a tidal breath at the points of zero flow on the P-V loop (end-inspiration or end-expiration).

What factors affect lung compliance?

> **Lung volume** – the slope of the P-V loop is not constant. It is steepest around FRC but then reduces at both low and high lung volumes (note that FRC is affected by many factors including age, body posture and body size, which will all in turn affect lung compliance).
> **Lung elasticity** – this is due to the elastin and collagen present in lung tissue. With ageing there is a gradual loss of elastic tissue and this increases compliance of the lungs. In emphysema, loss of elastin from lung tissue increases lung compliance. Compliance is reduced in pulmonary fibrosis due to increased collagen deposition in lung tissue and pulmonary congestion (e.g. oedema).
> **Surface tension** – this is the most important determinant of lung compliance. The water in alveolar fluid has a high surface tension and provides a force that tries to collapse the alveolus. Lung surfactant breaks up the surface tension of the fluid, increasing lung compliance and making the alveolus less likely to collapse. The effects of lack of pulmonary surfactant are clearly evident in conditions such as neonatal respiratory distress syndrome.

How can you calculate the work of breathing?

Mechanical work of breathing = Force × Distance
= Pressure × Volume

Thus, the work of breathing = cumulative product of pressure × volume of air moved over time

$$= \Delta P \times \Delta V / \Delta t$$

> During quiet breathing, most of the work performed is required to overcome elastic resistance (~65%). This inflates the lung and provides a store of elastic energy that gets released during expiration and is therefore viewed as 'useful' work. However, overcoming non-elastic resistance (e.g. airway resistance and viscosity, ~35%) results in energy being dissipated as heat and is viewed as 'wasted' work.
> The normal metabolic cost of breathing is approximately 0.5–1.0 mL O_2/L/min but this may increase to 2–4 mL O_2/L/min with hyperventilation. Work increases with increasing tidal volume, increasing respiratory flow and increasing airway resistance (e.g. COPD).

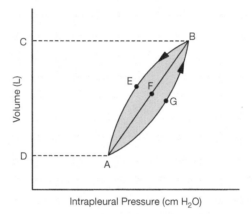

Fig. 10.2 Lung pressure-volume loop to show the work of breathing

> **Inspiration:** Work required to overcome the elastic recoil of the chest wall and lungs, airway resistance and viscosity (area AGBCD).
> **Expiration:** Expiratory work returned (area BEADC). This is passive under resting conditions and active during stress conditions.
> **Wasted work:** Area contained within the loop represents total wasted energy due to tissue and airway losses.

11. CONTROL OF RESPIRATION

Describe the control of respiration.

This is a straightforward question so keep it simple!

> Ventilation is regulated in order to maintain homeostasis of pH, PaO_2 and $PaCO_2$ in the blood.
> The respiratory centre is located in the brainstem and is composed of a group of nuclei within the medulla and pons.
> Three major brainstem respiratory neuronal areas have been identified:
>   • **Dorsal respiratory group (DRG) of neurons** – located in the medulla and controls inspiration
>   • **Pneumotaxic area** – located in the pons and assists in regulating inspiration
>   • **Ventral respiratory group (VRG) of neurons** – located in the medulla and regulates expiration.
> The respiratory centre receives input from higher CNS structures, peripheral and central chemoreceptors, and mechanoreceptors in the lungs and chest wall.

Brainstem

> DRG are mainly inspiratory neurons and control inspiration. This area has intrinsic automaticity and exhibits a ramp effect of increasing action potential frequency to the diaphragm (via the phrenic nerve, C3, 4, 5) and to the inspiratory muscles of the chest and abdomen (via intercostal nerves). They are responsible for basic ventilatory rhythm.
> Inspiration may be terminated prematurely by inhibitory impulses from the pneumotaxic centre. In effect, the pneumotaxic centre 'fine-tunes' inspiration.
> During normal quiet breathing expiration is passive. However, during exercise, for example the VRG of neurons are stimulated and drive the expiratory muscles.

Peripheral chemoreceptors

> Located in the aortic (near aortic arch) and carotid bodies (bifurcation of the common carotid artery). Cranial nerves X and IX link the receptors to the brainstem.
> The peripheral chemoreceptors primarily respond to hypoxia and respond to partial pressure of oxygen in the arterial blood rather than oxygen content of the blood. Thus patients with reduced blood oxygen content due to anaemia or carboxyhaemoglobin do not have respiratory stimulation via the peripheral chemoreceptors.
> The chemoreceptors are composed of glomus cells, which contain dopamine.
> Each carotid body receives an extremely high blood flow equivalent to $2 L/100 g$ tissue per minute.
> The aortic bodies respond to reductions in PaO_2 and rises in $PaCO_2$ by stimulating the inspiratory centre to increase respiratory rate.
> The carotid bodies respond not only to reductions in PaO_2 and rises in $PaCO_2$, but also to pH changes.
> Hypotension may also result in stimulation of the peripheral chemoreceptors probably via stagnant hypoxia.
> The respiratory stimulant doxapram acts via the peripheral chemoreceptors.
> Volatile anaesthetics abolish the peripheral chemoreceptor response to hypoxia.

Central chemoreceptors

> Situated in the ventral medulla, in an area that is extremely sensitive to hydrogen ions.
> Chemoreceptors are surrounded by extracellular fluid.
> When blood $PaCO_2$ rises, CO_2 diffuses across the blood–brain barrier into the CSF generating hydrogen ions [$CO_2 + H_2O \leftrightharpoons H_2CO_3 \leftrightharpoons H^+ + HCO_3^-$].
> pH thus falls (note that CSF has less protein than blood and therefore less buffering capacity) and this stimulates the inspiratory area.
> Hypercarbia provides an acute drive to increase ventilation for up to 48 hours; after this period CSF compensation occurs via increased HCO_3^- transport into the CSF in order to correct pH.

Voluntary control of respiration

> Cerebral cortex can override brainstem control, within limits, e.g. voluntary hyperventilation.

> Limbic system and hypothalamus – emotions such as rage and fear may also alter respiratory pattern.

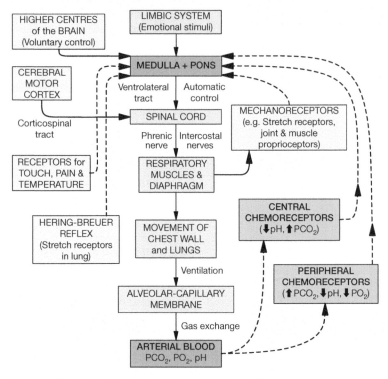

Fig. 11.1 Feedback systems involved in the control of respiration

Describe the response to inhalation of 5% CO_2 in oxygen.

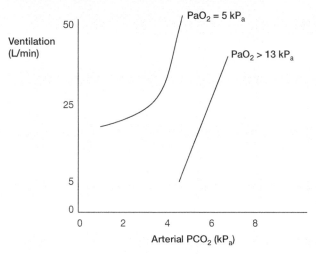

Fig. 11.2 Feedback systems involved in the control of respiration

> Over a short period of time, $PaCO_2$ will increase, which in turn will lead to an increase in CSF hydrogen ion concentration and thus a fall in pH which will be detected by the central chemoreceptors, leading to an increase in respiratory rate.
> An additional stimulus to respiration will come from the peripheral chemoreceptors, which will detect both the rise in $PaCO_2$ and the fall in pH, leading to input to the DRG of neurons via cranial nerves IX and X.
> Note that the ventilatory response to CO_2 is reduced by opiates, increasing age and sleep.

Describe the effects of raised CO_2 on the body.

> Hypercarbia stimulates respiration via activation of peripheral and central chemoreceptors.
> CVS – systemic vasodilatation, myocardial depression and arrhythmias.
> Pulmonary circulation – increased pulmonary vascular resistance. Respiratory acidosis.
> CNS – stimulates respiration but at high levels causes narcosis. Increases cerebral blood flow and intracranial pressure.
> Renal – slower compensation via bicarbonate retention and urinary hydrogen ion excretion.

Describe the ventilatory response to hypoxia.

> Hypoxaemia stimulates ventilation through its effects on the carotid and aortic bodies (peripheral chemoreceptors). Hypoxaemia is not a stimulus for the central chemoreceptors, although prolonged hypoxia will cause cerebral acidosis, which in turn can stimulate respiration.
> Isocapnic (holding CO_2 constant) oxygen curves illustrate the effect of changing PaO_2 on alveolar ventilation. The main stimulation of respiration through hypoxia occurs at $PaO_2 < 8\,kP_a$. Hypercarbia augments the ventilatory response to hypoxia.
> Increasing $PaCO_2$ by $0.1\,kP_a$ results in an increase in alveolar ventilation of approximately 1–2 L/min. In the same way a reduction in $PaCO_2$ results in a reduction in alveolar ventilation up until a $PaCO_2$ of $4\,kP_a$ below which there is no effect. Hypoxia produces a higher alveolar ventilation for any given $PaCO_2$.

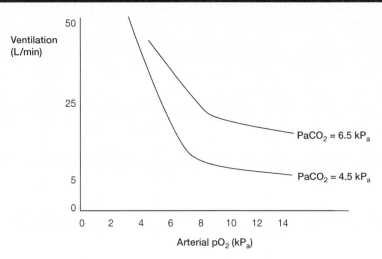

Fig. 11.3 Ventilatory response to PaO₂

12. ALTITUDE AND DIVING

Two extremes! The application of respiratory physiology principles to these two unusual environments requires a good understanding of the basic concepts of respiratory physiology and, therefore, is a popular examination question.

Altitude

The highest permanent habitation in the world is found in the Andes mountain range at 4877 m (16 000 ft) above sea level. In the northern Andes, the majority of inhabitants live above 2743 m (9000 ft). The capital cities of Bolivia (La Paz), Ecuador (Quito) and Colombia (Bogotá) are all high-altitude cities. La Paz is the highest capital city in the world at 3630 m (11 910 ft).

> Atmospheric pressure halves every 5500 m (18 000 ft).
> The percentage of oxygen in the atmosphere at sea level is about 21% and the barometric pressure is around 101 kP$_a$. As altitude increases, the percentage remains the same but the number of oxygen molecules per breath is reduced. At 3600 m (12 000 ft) the barometric pressure is only about 64 kP$_a$ (480 mmHg), so there are roughly 40% fewer oxygen molecules per breath thus the body must adjust to having less oxygen.
> At 19 200 m (63 000 ft) barometric pressure is 6.25 kP$_a$, meaning inspired PiO$_2$ is zero (as the partial pressure of water is 6.3 kP$_a$ and PiO$_2$ = FiO$_2$ × (P$_{atm}$ − P$_{H_2O}$)).

If a human being who resides at sea level were to be suddenly taken to the top of Mount Everest (8848 m/29 028 ft) he or she would succumb to hypoxia and lose consciousness. The body requires a period of acclimatisation during which physiological adaptation occurs in response to the relative lack of oxygen.

Describe the acute and chronic physiological responses to high altitude.

The alveolar gas equation is key to understanding the fundamental physiological response to high altitude:

$$P_AO_2 = PiO_2 - \frac{P_ACO_2}{R}$$

Where:

P$_A$O$_2$ Alveolar partial pressure of oxygen
PiO$_2$ Inspired pressure of oxygen = FiO$_2$ · (P$_{ATM}$ − P$_{H_2O}$)
P$_A$CO$_2$ Alveolar partial pressure of carbon dioxide (approximates with PaCO$_2$)
R   Respiratory quotient = CO$_2$ production / O$_2$ consumption (N=0.8).

> **Hyperventilation:** On ascent to altitude there is an increase in minute ventilation as a result of hypoxic stimulation of the peripheral chemoreceptors located in the aortic and carotid bodies. The hyperventilation results in a lowered arterial $PaCO_2$, which increases alveolar pressure of oxygen, as can be seen from the alveolar gas equation. The hypocarbia secondary to hyperventilation results in CSF alkalosis. However, this is transient as bicarbonate is excreted from the CSF over 24–48 hours and renally excreted.

> **Oxyhaemoglobin dissociation curve:** At moderate altitudes there is a right shift in the oxyhaemoglobin dissociation curve caused by increased levels of 2,3-DPG, thereby favouring oxygen unloading.
At high altitudes there is an overall left shift in the oxyhaemoglobin dissociation curve favouring oxygen uptake in the pulmonary capillaries.

> **Polycythaemia:** Increased erythropoietin secretion results in a slow increase in red cell count in order to increase oxygen-carrying capacity. However, this also results in a raised haematocrit, which can lead to thrombosis.

> **Cardiovascular responses:** Increase in heart rate and stroke volume from sympathetic stimulation from the effects of hypoxia in an attempt to maintain oxygen delivery to the tissues. Overall rise in myocardial work.

> **Hypoxic pulmonary vasoconstriction:** Results in an increase in pulmonary vascular resistance, which can lead to right heart failure.

> **Angiogenesis and enzyme changes:** Increase in capillary density with time, thereby reducing oxygen diffusion distance. This is associated with a change in intracellular oxidative enzymes favouring cellular respiration under hypoxic conditions.

How does high altitude affect volatile anaesthesia?

See Chapter 77, 'Vaporisers', for an in-depth explanation on this topic.

> Gas and vapour analysers measure partial pressure and assume sea level atmospheric pressure ($101\,kP_a$).
E.g. an oxygen analyser measuring $21\,kP_a$ will assume atmospheric pressure to be $101\,kP_a$ and provide a percentage of oxygen on the display of 21% or 0.21; however, if the analyser is used at an altitude where atmospheric pressure is only $70\,kP_a$, the analyser will under-read, displaying 21% when it should be 33%.

> TEC vaporisers function normally at altitude. The output of these vaporisers is a constant partial pressure of volatile agent *not* a constant volume percentage.
E.g. Vaporiser dialled to deliver 1% isoflurane:

  • Gas from the vaporising chamber is fully saturated with volatile agent (i.e. it has achieved its saturated vapour pressure (SVP) at that ambient temperature).

  • SVP is not affected by ambient pressure (i.e. does not change with altitude).

  • 1% isoflurane at sea level will have a partial pressure of 1%.

  • 1% isoflurane at altitude – the volatile agent from the vaporising chamber will be diluted into a less dense gas stream and therefore the concentration of isoflurane will be higher but the partial pressure remains the same as it would be at sea level. Clinical effect is dependent on the partial pressure and therefore remains the same.

What is acute mountain sickness (AMS)?

AMS is very common at high altitude. At over 3000 m (10 000 ft), 75% of people will have mild symptoms. The occurrence of AMS is dependent upon the elevation, the rate of ascent and individual susceptibility. Many people will experience mild AMS during the acclimatisation process. The symptoms usually start 12–24 hours after arrival at altitude and begin to decrease in severity around the third day. The symptoms of mild AMS include:

> Headache
> Nausea and dizziness
> Loss of appetite
> Fatigue
> Shortness of breath
> Disturbed sleep
> General feeling of malaise

What is high-altitude pulmonary oedema (HAPO)?

HAPO results from increased pulmonary extravascular lung water, which prevents effective oxygen exchange. As the condition progresses, severe hypoxaemia develops, which leads to cyanosis, impaired cerebral function and death. Symptoms of HAPO include:

> Shortness of breath at rest
> Tightness in the chest and a persistent cough bringing up white, watery or frothy fluid
> Marked fatigue and weakness
> A feeling of impending suffocation at night
> Confusion and irrational behaviour

What is high-altitude cerebral oedema (HACO)?

HACO is a potentially life-threatening complication of high altitude resulting from swelling of brain tissue secondary to fluid leakage. Symptoms of HACO include:

> Headache
> Weakness
> Disorientation
> Loss of coordination
> Decreasing levels of consciousness
> Loss of memory
> Hallucinations and psychotic behaviour
> Coma

Describe the treatment of AMS.

The only cure for mountain sickness is either acclimatisation or descent. Symptoms of mild AMS can be treated with analgesics for headache (e.g. ibuprofen), acetazolamide and dexamethasone.

> **Acetazolamide:** carbonic anhydrase inhibitor, which reduces bicarbonate formation and increases hydrogen ion concentration in the body, leading to development of a metabolic acidosis, which causes a respiratory compensation response resulting in an increase in minute ventilation and thus further lowering of $PaCO_2$.
> **Dexamethasone:** corticosteroid with predominantly glucocorticoid actions. It has anti-inflammatory properties and is useful in reducing cerebral oedema. Many pilgrims at the annual festival at Gosainkunda Lake in Nepal suffer from HACO following a rapid rate of ascent, and respond remarkably well to dexamethasone.

Other treatments for altitude sickness include the following

> **Nifedipine:** calcium channel blocker, most commonly used as an anti-hypertensive. It also has the effect of rapidly reducing pulmonary artery pressure by inhibiting hypoxic pulmonary vasoconstriction, thereby improving oxygen transfer. It can therefore be used to treat HAPO, though unfortunately its effectiveness is not anywhere as good as that of dexamethasone in HACO.
> **Furosemide:** loop diuretic, may be used to treat pulmonary oedema acutely. However, furosemide may also lead to collapse from low-volume shock if the victim is already dehydrated.
> **100% oxygen** also reduces the effects of altitude sickness.

Diving

During diving the opposite problems to altitude are seen. Barometric pressure increases by 1 atm for every 10 m descent (e.g. at a depth of 30 m barometric pressure will be 4 atm).

The following specific issues relate to respiratory physiology during diving:

> Effects of compression and decompression
> Inert gas narcosis
> Decompression sickness
> Oxygen toxicity
> High-pressure nervous syndrome

What mechanics are involved during compression and decompression?

During diving, as depth increases so too does barometric pressure. This increase in pressure is not a problem as long as it is balanced, i.e. there is no pressure gradient. Compression of gas-filled cavities such as the lungs, middle ear and sinuses will occur on descent. On rapid ascent the pressure difference between these cavities and barometric pressure may not have time to equilibrate, potentially resulting in complications such as pneumothoraces or perforated tympanic membranes.

What are the problems for scuba divers using an air mixture at depth?

Air contains 79% nitrogen. At high barometric pressures nitrogen has narcotic properties. This means that air can only be safely used up to a depth of 30–50 m.

At depths exceeding 50 m helium/oxygen gas mixtures are used. Helium does not exhibit the narcotic properties of nitrogen.

What limits the depth under water that a human can breathe via a snorkel?

A snorkel has an apparatus dead space, which means that if it is beyond a certain length, rebreathing of expired gas will occur, resulting in hypercarbia from impaired CO_2 elimination.

As the diver descends deeper under water, barometric pressure increases, which increases pressure within the circulation. However, because the diver's lungs are exposed to atmospheric pressure via the snorkel, a situation develops whereby pulmonary vascular pressure is greater than alveolar pressure, causing pulmonary oedema.

It becomes difficult to breathe via a snorkel at depths exceeding 1 m as a result of the compression effects on the chest.

Describe the physiology of decompression sickness.

> At depths exceeding 20 m nitrogen is absorbed into body tissues, especially fat. However, nitrogen has a low solubility and, therefore, equilibration between environment and body takes hours. If rapid ascent occurs, nitrogen comes out of solution forming bubbles. These bubbles can cause severe microvascular complications by obstructing blood flow; in the brain this can lead to visual disturbances or convulsions; joint pain can be severe.
> Treatment of decompression sickness is recompression, which forces nitrogen back into solution.
> Using a non-air gas mixture such as helium/oxygen reduces the risk of decompression sickness. Helium is 50% less soluble than nitrogen so less dissolves into tissues, reducing subsequent risk.
> As a rough rule of thumb it is safe for a diver to rapidly halve their ambient pressure, e.g. a rapid ascent from 10 m depth (2 atm) to the surface (1 atm).
> Commercial saturation divers who work at great depths live in high-pressure chambers so that their bodies remain saturated in nitrogen, thus avoiding decompression sickness. At the end of their period of diving they decompress, a process that will take a considerable amount of time!

What would happen if a diver performing a breath hold dive hyperventilated prior to the dive?

Competitive apnoea is an extreme sport in which competitors attempt to attain great depths, times or distances on a single breath without direct assistance of self-contained underwater breathing apparatus (scuba). The adaptations made by the human body while under water and at high pressure include:

> Bradycardia
> Vasoconstriction: redistribution of blood flow to myocardium, lungs and brain
> Splenic contraction

The record breath hold dive is 140 m. Hyperventilating prior to such a dive is not a sensible manoeuvre! Hyperventilation results in hypocarbia. The normal stimulus to terminate descent and commence ascent would be the development of hypoxia and hypercarbia. If the diver hyperventilated prior to such a dive, the only stimulus to ascend would be hypoxia. On ascent as barometric pressure falls so too would alveolar inspired oxygen (via alveolar gas equation), resulting in severe hypoxaemia and possible hypoxic seizures on ascent or even loss of consciousness.

Can oxygen toxicity develop during diving?

Yes.

> At oxygen partial pressure of greater than 2 atm oxygen toxicity is a risk; this equates to air diving at depths greater than 40 m (=5 atm / PO_2 > 2 atm). CNS excitation can lead to nausea, tinnitus, twitching and convulsions.
> The exact aetiology of the CNS toxicity from hyperoxia is not fully understood.

The implication for divers is the use of a hypoxic gas mixture to overcome this problem. For increasingly deep dives the oxygen concentration in the tank will be less than 21% and at extreme depths as low as 1%!

What is the physiological basis for hyperbaric oxygen therapy?

Increasing the arterial partial pressure of oxygen via increasing barometric pressure has a number of effects:

> Increases amount of dissolved oxygen
> Improves oxygen diffusion (Fick's law of diffusion)
> Promotes angiogenesis
> Improves function of polymorphs
> Inhibits growth of anaerobes (useful in gas gangrene)
> Displaces carbon monoxide from haemoglobin

At a barometric pressure of 3 atm there is sufficient dissolved oxygen alone to meet body oxygen requirements. This may be of use in a Jehovah's Witness patient with an acute perioperative anaemia refusing blood transfusion.

What are some of the clinical indications for hyperbaric oxygen therapy?

> **Gas lesions:** air or gas emboli and decompression sickness
> **Infections:** refractory osteomyelitis, necrotising soft tissue infections and clostridial infections
> **Global hypoxia:** carbon monoxide poisoning and severe anaemia
> **Regional hypoxia:** compromised grafts or free flaps, osteoradionecrosis and crush injuries.

What are the contraindications to hyperbaric oxygen therapy?

> Untreated pneumothorax
> Gas trapping in the lungs, e.g. lung bullae/bronchospasm
> Unusual drugs, e.g. doxorubicin

13. LUNG FUNCTION MEASUREMENT

How would you assess and measure a patient's lung function?

The aim of pre-operative lung function testing is to identify patients at high risk of perioperative pulmonary complications, in order to try and reduce these risks through patient preparation, targeted anaesthetic, and surgical techniques and planning for the appropriate level of post-operative care (e.g. HDU/ITU). If patient risk is high and the risk cannot be reduced, the risk–benefit ratio for surgery needs to be carefully evaluated and a decision has to be made as to whether to proceed.

Evaluation of a patient's pulmonary function requires correlation of history, examination findings and relevant investigation results in conjunction with the nature of proposed surgery.

Clinical

History and examination findings may provide valuable information about a patient's respiratory function. Pertinent history should include history of pre-existing lung disease (e.g. COPD, asthma, pulmonary fibrosis), smoking history (quantified via pack-year history), exercise tolerance, respiratory symptoms (cough, sputum production, wheeze), number and frequency of hospital admissions with respiratory problems, and current treatment regimen (e.g. bronchodilators, steroids, supplemental oxygen).

Risk factors for pulmonary complications include the following

Patient factors:
> Age >70 years
> History of lung disease
> BMI >30
> Smoking history >20-pack year

Surgical factors:
> Upper abdominal surgery
> Thoracic surgery
> Open vs. laparoscopic procedures

Investigations

Investigations should be targeted to the patient, i.e. based on clinical assessment and the nature of the planned surgery. Investigations that will have little or no clinical impact should be avoided. For example, a CXR in a 20-year-old ASA1 patient presenting for femoral hernia repair would be inappropriate. However, a CXR may well be indicated in a 20-year-old patient with cystic fibrosis presenting for the same procedure.

Peak expiratory flow rate (PEFR)

> Provides a simple method to measure airways obstruction, particularly in asthmatic patients.
> Normal range values are dependent on age, sex and height.
>> 20-year-old female height 1.60 m PEFR 433 L/min
>> 20-year-old male height 1.83 m PEFR 654 L/min

Arterial blood gas (ABG) analysis

> Allows evaluation of gas exchange by providing essential information about the state of oxygenation, acid–base balance, chronicity and severity of respiratory failure.
> It is useful to have baseline arterial blood gases, especially for patients undergoing surgery, where there will inevitably be perioperative changes in gas exchange, as it allows for easier interpretation of these subsequent changes.

Spirometry

> This is the timed measurement of dynamic lung volumes during forced expiration and inspiration.
> Measurements – forced vital capacity (FVC), forced expiratory volume in one second (FEV1) and the ratio of these two volumes (FEV1/FVC).
> Measurement of maximum expiratory flow over the middle 50% of the vital capacity (FEF25–75%) is a sensitive index of small airway function.
> Measurements of forced maximal flow during expiration and inspiration flow can be made as a function of volume thus generating a flow volume loop, the shape of which also contains information of diagnostic value.

Interpretation of spirometry data

> The presence of ventilatory abnormality can be implied if any of FEV1, FVC or FEV1/VC ratios are outside the reference ranges.
> Interrelationships of the various measurements are important diagnostically:
>   • FEV1/FVC <80% constitutes an obstructive ventilatory defect (e.g. asthma/COPD)
>   • FEV1/FVC >80% constitutes a restrictive ventilatory defect (e.g. pulmonary fibrosis/kyphoscoliosis).
> It is routine practice to quantify the degree of reversibility of an obstructive defect by measuring spirometry before and after the administration of a bronchodilator. Generally, an improvement in FEV1 of 200 mL or more infers significant reversibility if the baseline FEV1 is <1.5 L, as does an improvement of >15% if the FEV1 is >1.5 L.

Flow volume loops

> Constructed from spirometric data. Note that expiratory flow is above the x-axis, whereas inspiratory flow is represented below the x-axis.
> Analysis of the flow volume loops can be diagnostic (*see* Fig. 13.1).

Cardiopulmonary exercise testing (CPET)

> Non-invasive and objective method of evaluating both cardiac and pulmonary functions.
> Cycle ergometry is the most common mode of exercise.
> Safe procedure, with a risk of death between 2 and 5 per 100 000 exercise tests performed.
> Computerised test provides a breath-by-breath analysis of respiratory gas exchange at rest and during a period of exercise, the intensity of which is increased incrementally until symptoms limit testing or the patient reaches maximal levels.
> Information on airflow, O_2 consumption, CO_2 production and heart rate is collected and used for computation of other variables such as oxygen uptake and the anaerobic threshold.
> Primarily determines if the patient has normal or reduced maximal exercise capacity ($\dot{V}O_2$ max). Reduced $\dot{V}O_2$ max can further suggest probable causes.
> Used to define which organ systems (pulmonary or cardiac) contribute to a patient's symptoms of exertional dyspnoea and exercise intolerance and to what extent.
> The anaerobic threshold may also be measured using CPET.
> More sensitive for detecting early or subclinical disease and is establishing a key role in pre-operative assessment of high-risk patients undergoing major surgery.

Respiratory muscle strength	> Assessed globally by measurement of maximum mouth pressures. Maximum inspiratory mouth pressure measurements reflect the force-generating capacity of inspiratory muscles.
	> Measurements are taken during maximum inspiratory effort against an occlusion at residual volume (where mechanical advantage of inspiratory muscles is greatest) or at FRC.
Carbon monoxide diffusing capacity (DLco or transfer factor)	> Measure of the ability of gas to transfer from alveoli to red blood cells across the alveolar epithelium and the capillary endothelium.
	> Depends not only on the area and thickness of the blood–gas barrier but also on the volume of blood in the pulmonary capillaries. The distribution of alveolar volume and ventilation also affects the measurement.
	> Measured by sampling end-expiratory gas for carbon monoxide (CO) after a patient inspires a small amount of CO, holds their breath and exhales.
	> Measured DLco should be adjusted for alveolar volume (which is estimated from dilution of helium) and the patient's haematocrit.
	> DLco is reported as mL/min/mmHg and as a percentage of a predicted value.
Conditions that are associated with a reduced DLco	> Primary pulmonary hypertension
	> Pulmonary embolism
	> Emphysema
	> Pulmonary fibrosis
Conditions that are associated with an increased DLco	> Polycythaemia
	> Alveolar haemorrhage

Within the perioperative context of lung function assessment, it should be remembered that the input of a respiratory physician might be invaluable.

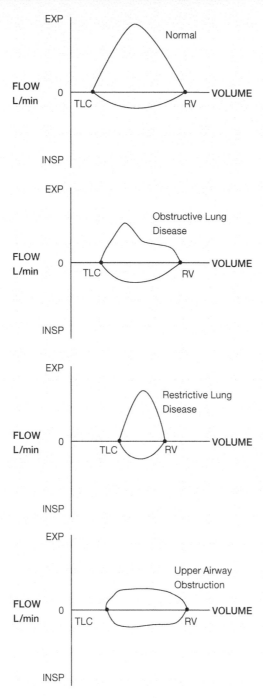

Fig. 13.1 Flow volume loops in different disease states

14. EFFECTS OF ANAESTHESIA ON LUNG FUNCTION

Can you describe the effects of general anaesthesia on lung function?

General anaesthesia has multiple important effects on lung function. The easiest way to think of the changes is to divide them into categories:

Respiratory control
> The patient's basal metabolic rate drops by 15% following induction of anaesthesia, due to thalamic inhibition.
> The response to hypercapnia is blunted and the acute responses to acidosis and hypoxia are almost entirely abolished.

Lung mechanics
> Following induction, functional residual capacity (FRC) falls by 15–20% because there is a loss of muscle tone. This decreased tone reduces the bucket handle action of the rib cage, which consequently moves less; breathing is more dependent on the movement of the diaphragm, which is similarly weakened. Phasic activity develops in the expiratory muscles, which are normally silent.
> In spontaneous, awake ventilation, expiration is a passive movement; under anaesthesia it becomes an active one.
> Lung compliance is reduced and airway resistance increases slightly; these combine to increase the work of breathing.
> Mucociliary transport mechanisms are reduced, which can cause retention of secretions.

Gas exchange
> The changes described above can cause atelectasis and inhibit hypoxic pulmonary vasoconstriction. Logically, the application of PEEP should improve the situation as it helps to 'splint' the alveoli open. However, applying PEEP will also reduce blood flow to the splinted areas, by altering the pressure across the alveoli and therefore capillary walls (remember Starling's resistors and West's zones of the lung). So PEEP may actually increase $\dot{V}/\dot{Q}$ mismatching and should be applied with care in unstable patients. As with all things, this is a balance of risk. The application of PEEP may also destabilise the cardiovascular system in a particularly sick patient. Without the application of any PEEP, around 10% of pulmonary blood is shunted or perfuses areas with low $\dot{V}/\dot{Q}$
> Alveolar dead space rises from 0 to 70 mL and physiological dead space from 150 to 220 mL. Intubation decreases dead space, but this effect is reduced by connectors etc.

All the changes described are exaggerated in those patients with lung disease.

Smokers should be counselled to stop smoking at least 6 weeks prior to their operations to allow their mucociliary and inflammatory cell function to return to somewhere approaching normal. Failing this, they should definitely not smoke for at least 12 hours prior to surgery, as the half-life of carbon monoxide is 4 hours.

In all patients, the effects of anaesthesia on lung function will last a few hours post-operatively. After major surgery, or in those with lung disease, the effects may last many days.

If the patient is placed on their side on the table, how will their position affect the flow of gases into the lungs?

> The flow of gases is dependent upon whether the patient is spontaneously breathing or being ventilated with positive pressure.
> If the patient is spontaneously ventilating, gas will be drawn into the dependent lung, i.e. the lowermost lung. The situation is reversed, however, when the patient is ventilated. Now gas will follow the path of least resistance into the non-dependent lung, whose total compliance would be greater as it does not have the weight of the thorax pressing down on it. As blood is preferentially distributed to the lower lung, this can cause $\dot{V}/\dot{Q}$ mismatching and desaturation.

It is easy to remember which way round this is as it is obvious that blood will preferentially perfuse the dependent lung under the influence of gravity. In our natural state, e.g. asleep in bed on our side, nature would not invent a system that would worsen oxygenation – so the air must also flow into the dependent lung to increase $\dot{V}/\dot{Q}$ matching. A practical application of this principle can be seen in ITU when we see patients improve/desaturate as they are turned and the good/bad lung is preferentially ventilated.

Table 14.1 Summary of distribution (%) of ventilation under anaesthesia in the lateral position:

	Dependent Lung	Non-dependent Lung
Awake, spontaneously breathing	60%	40%
GA, spontaneously breathing	45%	55%
GA, IPPV	40%	60%
Thoracotomy	30%	70%

15. BARORECEPTORS AND CONTROL OF BLOOD PRESSURE

What types of baroreceptor are there?

Baroreceptors are mechanoreceptors that respond to stretch and are also known as stretch or pressure receptors. They are terminal myelinated nerve endings, located within vessel walls and the cardiac chambers. Their action potential firing rate is altered in response to changes in blood pressure, which creates a negative feedback mechanism responsible for the autonomic regulation of blood pressure.

They may be classified as high- or low-pressure baroreceptors:

> **High-pressure arterial baroreceptors:** Located within the walls of the aortic arch and carotid sinus (a small dilatation of the internal carotid artery just above its bifurcation). Because of their proximity to blood leaving the heart, these receptors are well positioned to control perfusion pressures to the coronary and cerebral circulations. They are involved in the rapid short-term control of blood pressure.
> **Low-pressure baroreceptors:** Located in the chambers of the heart, large systemic veins and the pulmonary vasculature. These receptors bring about changes in blood volume and are involved in the slower and sustained control of blood pressure.

How do the high-pressure baroreceptors work?

> The aortic arch and carotid sinus baroreceptors discharge impulses along the vagus and glossopharyngeal nerves, respectively, to the nucleus tractus solitarius in the medulla. Here, the vasomotor and cardio-inhibitory centres modulate sympathetic and parasympathetic outflow, in turn restoring blood pressure towards normal.
> As blood pressure rises, the rate of discharge along these nerves increases, leading to a reduction in sympathetic outflow and increase in parasympathetic transmission. The consequent reduction in blood vessel tone, heart rate and contractility leads to a reduction in blood pressure (MAP = SV × HR × SVR). Conversely, the rate of discharge decreases with reductions in blood pressure, leading to increased sympathetic outflow.
> As this system relies on neural transmission, it is extremely fast and is responsible for the beat-to-beat control of blood pressure. For example, these baroreceptors mediate the bradycardia, which is sometimes observed in patients following administration of a bolus dose of vasopressor such as phenylephrine.
> Although high-pressure baroreceptors respond to both a rise and a fall in blood pressure, their most important role is in response to a fall (e.g. haemorrhage, standing up).

What reflexes are elicited by a rapid fall in blood pressure, e.g. sudden 2 L blood loss?	The physiological response involves cardiovascular, neurohumoral and renal compensatory mechanisms

> **Baroreceptor reflex activation – immediate response**
>   • Reduced baroreceptor (aortic arch and carotid sinus) input due to reduced vessel stretch leads to reduced afferent discharge in glossopharyngeal and vagus nerves. Cardio-inhibitory centre is inhibited while the vasomotor centre is activated, leading to reduced parasympathetic activity and increased sympathetic activity, resulting in increased force of cardiac contraction, tachycardia and increased SVR.
> **Cardiovascular**
>   • Redistribution of cardiac output from skin, muscle and viscera to brain and heart.
> **Hypothalamic–Pituitary–Adrenal responses**
>   • Increased ADH secretion from the posterior pituitary, leading to water conservation
>   • Increased adrenal release of noradrenaline, adrenaline and cortisol via sympathetic nervous system activation
> **Starling's forces**
>   • Favour interstitial fluid movement into the circulation through a fall in intravascular hydrostatic pressure and a rise in oncotic pressure
> **Renin–Angiotensin–Aldosterone system**
>   • Fall in renal blood flow, detected by juxtaglomerular apparatus, leads to release of renin, which converts angiotensinogen to angiotensin I. Angiotensin converting enzyme (ACE) secreted by the lungs and kidneys converts this into angiotensin 2, which causes vasoconstriction and stimulates the release of aldosterone.
>   • Aldosterone increases sodium and water re-absorption at the distal convoluted tubules, thereby expanding plasma volume.

What is the Bainbridge reflex?

Also known as the atrial reflex. A rapid increase in venous return to the heart (e.g. rapid IV fluid bolus) may lead to activation of low-pressure atrial stretch receptors, resulting in an increase in heart rate. The purpose of the tachycardia is to restore atrial (and vena caval) pressures to normal by removing blood volume from the right atrium. The Bainbridge reflex is involved in respiratory sinus arrhythmia where heart rate momentarily increases with inspiration (lower intrathoracic pressure) due to increased venous return.

What is the Bezold–Jarisch reflex?

Activation of left ventricular chemo- and baroreceptors, located in the left ventricle, results in unopposed parasympathetic tone, leading to the triad of bradycardia, vasodilation and hypotension. This is known synonymously as vasovagal syncope, neurocardiogenic syncope or the Bezold–Jarisch reflex. It is triggered by reduced venous return to the heart, but may also have an affective component, e.g. pain or fear. Situations relevant to anaesthesia include regional anaesthesia (spinal, epidural and interscalene blocks where sympathetic output is blocked), haemorrhage/hypovolaemia and inferior vena cava compression in supine pregnant patients. Treatment is by restoring venous return with fluids and administration of sympathomimetics, in particular ephedrine. This reflex may also explain the bradycardia associated with acute postero-inferior myocardial infarction, thrombolysis, coronary angiography and exertion syncope seen in aortic stenosis.

Describe the physiological control of blood pressure.

Blood pressure regulation occurs not only from beat to beat but also in the longer term over months to years. Mean arterial pressure is the product of cardiac output (heart rate × stroke volume) and systemic vascular resistance.

$$MAP = CO \times SVR$$

> **Short-term regulation:** Mediated largely by the arterial and cardiac baroreceptors and the vasomotor centre in the nucleus tractus solitarius, which ultimately alter the balance between parasympathetic and sympathetic discharge, thereby altering heart rate, stroke volume and systemic vascular resistance.

> **Long-term regulation:** Mediated by neurohumoral, renal, metabolic, race and genetic factors. The following factors may all affect long-term blood pressure:
> - Sodium intake
> - Atrial natriuretic peptide
> - Bradykinin
> - Nitric oxide
> - Glucocorticoids
> - Renal function
> - Psychological stress
> - Obesity – with a possible link to insulin resistance
> - Atherosclerosis
> - Renin – angiotensin – aldosterone system

16. CARDIAC CYCLE

This is a core topic and a common examination question. Make sure you are able to draw the cardiac cycle and explain the pressure changes and events during each of the five phases.

Describe the pressure changes that occur during the cardiac cycle.

Describe the five phases of the cardiac cycle.

Phase 1: atrial contraction
Phase 2: ventricular isovolumetric contraction
Phase 3: ventricular ejection
Phase 4: ventricular isovolumetric relaxation
Phase 5: passive ventricular filling.

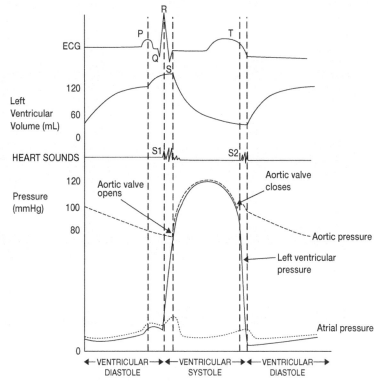

Fig. 16.1 The cardiac cycle

17. CORONARY CIRCULATION

Describe the coronary circulation.

> The arterial blood supply to the heart comes from the right coronary artery (RCA) and the left coronary artery (LCA), which arise from the anterior and posterior aortic sinuses respectively.
> The RCA supplies the right atrium, right ventricle, sinoatrial node and, in 90% of people, also the atrioventricular node.
> The LCA divides into the left anterior descending (LAD) artery and the left circumflex (LCx) artery and supplies the left atrium, left ventricle and most of the interventricular septum.
> In 30% of the population the LCA and RCA supply equal proportions of blood while in 50% the RCA is the dominant vessel.
> Venous drainage occurs predominantly via the coronary sinus. This receives blood from the great cardiac vein (draining the anterior aspect of the heart) and the middle cardiac vein (draining the posterior aspect of the heart). In addition, there are other vessels that drain directly into the heart chambers including the thebesian veins, which contribute towards true shunt.

What is autoregulation?

> Autoregulation refers to the intrinsic ability of an organ to maintain a constant blood flow despite a varying perfusion pressure. The heart, kidney and brain are all examples of organs that exhibit this ability.

How is coronary blood flow autoregulated?

> The heart can autoregulate its blood supply at coronary perfusion pressures (CoPP) between 60 and 180 mmHg. Outside this range, the coronary circulation becomes pressure dependent.

Autoregulation occurs via a combination of the following mechanisms:

Metabolic: During periods of increased myocardial activity, local tissue hypoxia and increased metabolic waste products such as H^+, K^+, adenosine and CO_2 cause vasodilatation of the coronary vessels, thereby increasing coronary blood flow.

Myogenic: When the pressure within a small artery or arteriole is increased, the smooth muscle within these vessels automatically constricts, thereby reducing blood flow. The reverse happens when the pressure within these vessels falls.

Endothelial: Vascular endothelium produces various vasoactive substances including nitric oxide (NO), endothelium-derived relaxing factor (EDRF) and prostacyclin (PGI_2), all of which produce vasodilatation; conversely endothelin and thromboxane A_2 produce vasoconstriction. When endothelium is damaged (e.g. atherosclerotic plaques or ischaemia) the production of these vasoactive substances is reduced, making coronary vessels prone to vasospasm and platelet aggregation.

Autonomic: ANS exerts a weak effect on the coronary circulation. α-adrenergic receptor stimulation causes vasoconstriction while β-adrenergic and vagal stimulation leads to vasodilatation of coronary vessels.

Hormonal: Vasoactive hormones require an intact endothelium in order to produce their effect. Atrial natriuretic peptide causes vasodilatation while vasopressin and angiotensin II cause vasoconstriction.

What factors affect myocardial oxygen supply?

Myocardial oxygen supply is determined by coronary blood flow and the arterial oxygen content (CaO_2).

Determinants of coronary blood flow:

Coronary perfusion pressure (CoPP = Aortic pressure – Intraventricular pressure). During systole the CoPP of the left ventricle can equal zero (or less) and therefore coronary blood flow only occurs during diastole.

In systole:

$$LVCoPP = [SBP - LVESP] = [120\,mmHg - 120\,mmHg] = 0\,mmHg$$

In diastole:

$$LVCoPP = [DBP - LVEDP] = [70\,mmHg - 10\,mmHg] = 60\,mmHg.$$

However, the coronary blood flow to both atria and the right ventricle occurs throughout the cardiac cycle.

In systole:

$$RVCoPP = [SBP - RVESP] = [120 - 25] = 95\,mmHg$$

In diastole:

$$RVCoPP = [DBP - RVEDP] = [70 - 5] = 65\,mmHg.$$

Perfusion time: As the heart rate increases, the diastolic time and therefore the coronary perfusion time, especially to the left ventricle, is reduced.

Coronary vessel patency: Atherosclerotic vessels are stenosed and have a reduced blood flow (as indicated by the Hagen–Poiseuille formula).

Coronary vessel diameter: The wider the diameter, the greater the blood flow (hence the administration of GTN in angina).

Blood viscosity: Haematocrit is a major determinant of blood viscosity and from the Hagen–Poiseuille formula it can be seen that as viscosity increases, flow decreases. However, as haematocrit decreases, so does the oxygen-carrying capacity of blood.

Determinants of arterial oxygen content:

$$CaO_2 = [Hb \times Sats \times 1.34] + [PaO_2 \times 0.023]$$

From this equation it can be seen that the only parameters we can manipulate are the Hb and the PaO_2 (see Chapter 4, 'Oxygen transport', for full explanation of the above equation).

What are the major determinants of myocardial oxygen consumption?

The heart has the highest oxygen consumption per tissue mass of any organ in the body, requiring 10 mL O_2/min/100 g at rest and 70 mL/min/100 g during heavy exercise (the kidney uses 5 mL/min/100 g while the brain uses 3 mL/min/100 g). As a result, the heart receives 5% of the cardiac output, giving it a coronary blood flow of 250 mL/min.

In order to support such high oxygen consumption, the heart at rest extracts approximately 70% of its coronary blood oxygen content (remember that the rest of the body only extracts, on average 25%, of its arterial O_2 content). Therefore, during periods of increased mechanical activity the only way the heart can meet its increased oxygen consumption is by increasing its coronary blood flow.

Factors that determine myocardial oxygen consumption include heart rate, contractility, afterload, tissue mass and temperature (cold cardioplegic solutions are used during cardiopulmonary bypass surgery to reduce myocardial oxygen consumption and minimise risk of ischaemia).

18. EXERCISE

The physiological response to exercise involves primarily cardio-respiratory and metabolic adaptations. The exact physiological response is determined not only by the intensity and duration of exercise but also by the underlying level of fitness of the individual.

Describe the physiological changes that occur in response to exercise.

In healthy individuals, predictable physiological changes occur during exercise.

At rest, oxygen consumption is approximately 250 mL/min. During strenuous exercise oxygen consumption may rise to over 4000 mL/min. This massive increase in oxygen consumption requires a cardio-respiratory response to increase oxygen delivery.

Respiratory changes:

On initiation of exercise, minute ventilation increases dramatically from a basal rate of approximately 5 L/min to over 20 L/min via a combination of increase in respiratory rate and tidal volume. This initial increase is thought to occur in response to afferent impulses from proprioceptors in muscle.

As exercise progresses, minute ventilation continues to rise linearly with work rate and may reach in excess of 150 L/min.

Oxygen consumption also increases linearly with work rate, until the subject reaches their $\dot{V}O_2$ max, at which point it becomes constant.

$\dot{V}O_2$ max is the maximum amount of oxygen a subject can utilise at a cellular level to produce ATP to power the exercise. It is measured in mL/kg/min.

$\dot{V}O_2$ max is the best and most reproducible index of cardiopulmonary fitness. Any increase in work rate above $\dot{V}O_2$ max can only occur via anaerobic glycolysis.

Minimal changes occur in arterial pH, $PaCO_2$ and PaO_2 during exercise.

Cardiovascular changes:

Cardiac output increases as a consequence of a rise in heart rate and augmentation of stroke volume because of increased force of systolic contraction. These chronotropic and inotropic effects on the heart are the result of activation of the sympathetic nervous system and a rise in LVEDP resulting from increased venous return from muscle and capacitance beds. In trained athletes, the left ventricle hypertrophies and a resting bradycardia is often present. Trained athletes may achieve cardiac outputs in excess of 30 L/min during exercise.

Muscle blood flow is increased during exercise as a consequence of accumulation of metabolites such as adenosine and potassium. Consequently, SVR is reduced. Oxygen extraction by the muscle is also increased during exercise.

The oxyhaemoglobin dissociation curve is shifted to the right because of the reduced local pH in exercising muscle and the increased temperature. Blood is also redistributed to the skin to enable heat loss.

What metabolic changes occur during exercise?

The primary source of fuel to produce energy in the early stages of exercise is carbohydrate, stored as glycogen and liberated into glucose. The metabolism of carbohydrate is described in Chapter 19 'Carbohydrate metabolism'.

As glycogen stores become depleted during prolonged exercise, the metabolic substrate switches to fatty acids. If fat is fully oxidised via the Krebs cycle it leads to the generation of 129 molecules of ATP. The rate of ATP re-synthesis from fat is too slow to be of great importance during high-intensity exercise such as sprinting however it is important during endurance exercise.

Under normal circumstances protein metabolism does not contribute to ATP generation because it is an essential structural component of the body. However, in extreme conditions (e.g. ultra marathon runners or starvation) protein can be used to generate ATP.

What is the anaerobic threshold (AT)?

The AT marks the onset of anaerobic metabolism as a result of inadequate oxygen delivery. At this point lactate begins to accumulate in the blood. The $\dot{V}O_2$ at this point is called the anaerobic threshold. It is measured in mL/Kg/min of O_2. The anaerobic threshold typically occurs between 45% and 65% of the $\dot{V}O_2$ max in healthy untrained individuals and generally does not exceed 80% even in endurance-trained athletes.

Training can result in an increase in both $\dot{V}O_2$ max and anaerobic threshold.

What is the respiratory exchange ratio (RER)?

The RER is the ratio of CO_2 production to O_2 consumption:

$$RER = \dot{V}CO_2/\dot{V}O_2$$

The RER represents the metabolic exchange of gases in the body's tissues and is dependent in part on the predominant fuel (carbohydrate vs. fat) used for cellular metabolism.

At rest and with early exercise, the $\dot{V}CO_2$ curve runs slightly below the $\dot{V}O_2$ curve (RER 0.8) but once the anaerobic threshold is passed, additional non-metabolic CO_2 is produced, resulting in a steep rise in $\dot{V}CO_2$ and an accompanying rise in the RER, ultimately exceeding 1.0.

19. CARBOHYDRATE METABOLISM

A question on carbohydrate metabolism can make even the most stoical candidate's heart sink. The subject is potentially vast and it seems to consist of a meaningless lists of indecipherable molecules being phosphorylated, broken down and then put back together again! Luckily, a basic overview should be enough to get you through. We have tried to pull out the salient points below.

Explain the pathways involved in metabolising a glucose load.

Carbohydrates are organic molecules made up of carbon, hydrogen and oxygen. They are consumed in the diet as either simple sugars (glucose and fructose) or complex sugars (starch and cellulose). Complex sugars are essentially simple sugars assembled into chains for ease of storage (e.g. starch from plants, glycogen from animals), or to form structures (e.g. cellulose in plants).

During the digestive process, which starts in the mouth with mastication, complex sugars are broken down into simple sugars that can be transported across cell walls and used to make energy in the form of ATP. The simple sugar glucose is the body's most readily available energy source and can be used by all cells.

The main pathways in glucose metabolism are:

Glycolysis:
This umbrella term describes the generation of ATP from glucose molecules. It can be divided into three stages, which will be considered in turn:

- Glycolysis
- The Krebs cycle
- Oxidative phosphorylation and the electron transport chain

Gluconeogenesis:
The generation of glucose from substrates such as pyruvate.

Glycogenesis:
The synthesis of glycogen to store glucose.

Glycogenolysis:
The breakdown of glycogen to liberate glucose.

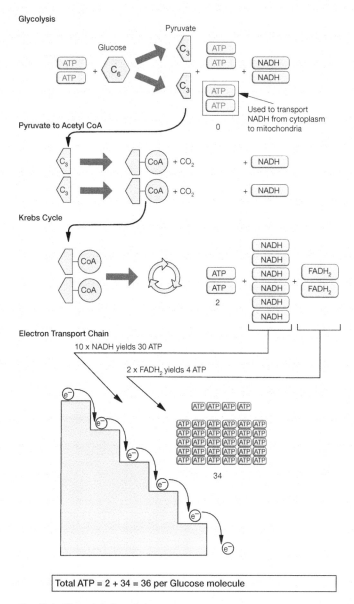

Glycolysis

Pyruvate

Glucose

Pyruvate to Acetyl CoA

$+ CO_2$

$+ CO_2$

Krebs Cycle

Used to transport NADH from cytoplasm to mitochondria

Electron Transport Chain

10 x NADH yields 30 ATP

2 x FADH$_2$ yields 4 ATP

Total ATP = 2 + 34 = 36 per Glucose molecule

Fig. 19.1   The metabolism of glucose

Glycolysis

The aim of glycolysis is to split the 6-carbon sugar glucose into two molecules of the 3-carbon sugar pyruvate. This is achieved by phosphorylation of the glucose molecule, using the phosphate from one ATP molecule. Following this, glucose-6-phosphate is converted to fructose-6-phosphate (a 5-carbon sugar) by phosphofructokinase. This molecule is then phosphorylated again to form fructose-1,6-bisphosphate, using the phosphate from another ATP molecule. This molecule is then split in two, and a series of further reactions lead to the formation of a two-pyruvate molecules (one from each half of the cleaved fructose-1,6,bisphosphate). Two molecules of ATP are formed as a result of the generation of each pyruvate molecule. So, from each molecule of glucose, glycolysis generates four ATPs while two are used up, making a net gain of two ATPs.

Anaerobic vs aerobic respiration

When oxygen supply is inadequate, pyruvate will enter an **anaerobic pathway**. In this pathway, pyruvate is converted into lactate (also called lactic acid). Each pyruvate molecule that enters this pathway will generate one ATP and, since two pyruvates are produced from each molecule of glucose, this gives a net gain of two ATPs from this stage of the pathway.

This is clearly not much compared to aerobic respiration, but it is better than nothing and it keeps the conversion of glucose to pyruvate going by reducing the concentration of pyruvate in the cells.

Cells that lack mitochondria, e.g. red blood cells, must respire anaerobically at all times.

When the oxygen supply is adequate, pyruvate will enter the **aerobic pathway**, the Krebs cycle.

The Krebs cycle

This is also called the citric acid cycle or the tricarboxylic acid (TCA) cycle.

To enter the Krebs cycle, pyruvate is transported into the mitochondria where it is converted into the 2-carbon molecule, acetyl coenzyme A (acetyl CoA) by pyruvate dehydrogenase. Acetyl CoA enters the Krebs cycle by being bound to the 4-carbon molecule oxaloacetate to form the 6-carbon molecule, citrate. This molecule is then broken down again to a 5-carbon molecule and again to back to oxaloacetate and so on (hence the cycle…).

During this cycle, molecules that are high in energy are generated and each turn of the cycle yields:

- 1 ATP
- 3 NADH (nicotinamide adenine dinucleotide. NAD^+ is a coenzyme that acts as an electron acceptor to create NADH)
- 1 $FADH_2$ (flavin adenine dinucleotide is a redox cofactor, i.e. it undergoes reduction-oxidation)

The cycle will turn twice for each molecule of glucose metabolised.

Oxidative phosphorylation and the electron transport chain

The electron transport chain uses the NADH and $FADH_2$ generated in the Krebs cycle to make ATP. In a series of enzymatic reactions that occur at the inner mitochondrial membrane, electrons from NADH and FAD_2 are transferred repeatedly from donor (e.g. NADH) to acceptor (e.g. oxygen) molecules further down the 'chain'. This process is coupled with the transfer of H^+ ions across the inner mitochondrial membrane and this sets up a concentration gradient across the membrane. H^+ ions then flow back across the membrane through ATP synthase channels and in doing so supply the energy needed to phosphorylate ADP to produce ATP.

When they come to the end of the electron transport chain, the electrons are accepted by oxygen molecules, which go on to combine with H^+ ions to form water. Without oxygen, the electrons cannot keep being passed down the chain and respiration ceases.

For each molecule of glucose, the electron transport chain yields **34 ATP**.

Gluconeogenesis

Gluconeogenesis describes the synthesis of glucose from:

- Pyruvate
- Lactate
- Glycerol
- Alanine and glutamine (amino acids)

This process exists in case the supply of dietary glucose runs out. The brain preferentially uses glucose as its fuel source, although it can use ketones to some degree, and so it is vital that there are alternative sources of this substrate.

Gluconeogenesis takes place mainly in the liver, and to a small extent, in the kidneys. Turning **pyruvate** into glucose is not simply the reverse of glycolysis, instead pyruvate (3-carbon) is converted to oxaloacetate (4-carbon) at the expense of one ATP molecule. From here oxaloacetate is converted to phosphoenolpyruvate by the enzyme phosphoenolpyruvate carboxykinase, and from then a series of reactions generate glucose.

The net cost of synthesising glucose from pyruvate is 6 ATPs, but these glucose can then be fed back into the glycolysis pathway to yield 36 ATPs.

Lactate produced in times of anaerobic respiration, can be converted into pyruvate and back to glucose in the liver in the Cori cycle (also called the lactic acid cycle). Lactate can be used as a substrate by some tissues.

Amino acids can provide a source of energy because during the process of their metabolism many intermediary products are formed and broken down and many of these can be fed into the Krebs cycle, e.g. pyruvate, acetyl CoA, oxaloacetate, α ketoglutarate, to yield ATP. This fuel source becomes more significant during starvation, when muscle will be broken down to fuel respiration.

Glycerol is liberated when triglycerides (fat) are hydrolysed to fatty acids and glycerol. These fatty acids then undergo β oxidation into acetyl CoA, which is fed into the Krebs cycle. The glycerol released is fed directly into the Krebs cycle as dihydroxyacetone phosphate. Fat yields approximately 9 kcal/g compared to 4 kcal/g from carbohydrate though the process of liberating the energy is much slower. Even very slim people have significant fat reserves, which will act as an energy source when carbohydrates are exhausted.

Glycogenesis

Glucose is stored as the multi-branched polysaccharide glycogen, primarily in the liver and muscles. Glycogenesis occurs when glucose and ATP are present in relatively high amounts as it uses up one ATP molecule for every glucose molecule incorporated into the chain. Glucose is stored in glycogen as glucose-6-phosphate.

Glycogenolysis

Glycogen is broken down to release glucose during glycogenolysis. This process involves the removal of glucose monomers from the storage chain by phosphorylation. The reaction is catalysed by glycogen phosphorylase. A series of further steps result in glucose-6-phosphate being fed into the glycolysis pathway.

Glycogen stored in the liver is broken down by glycolysis, which releases glucose into the blood for utilisation by other cells, while that present in the skeletal muscle provides an immediate energy source for muscle contraction.

Glycogen provides a source of energy that can be mobilised instantly. However, it is limited and, during intense exercise, the store will be exhausted in around 3–4 hours.

Regulation of glycogen synthesis is reciprocal. The following act via G-protein-coupled receptors to exert their effects:

- Adrenaline – stimulates glycolysis
- Glucagon – stimulates glycolysis and inhibits glycogenesis
- Insulin – inhibits glycolysis and stimulates glycogenesis.

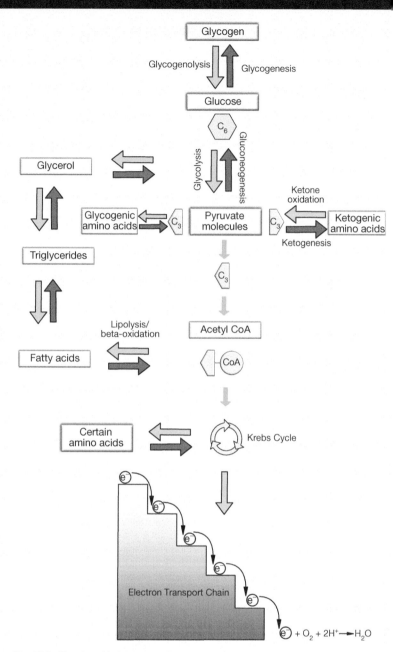

Fig. 19.2 Overview of fuel sources

20. STARVATION

Many patients admitted to hospital experience poor nutritional intake either as a direct result of their disease process or because of poor oral intake. Starvation has clinically important effects on the body and the physiological and biochemical adaptations that occur in response to starvation lend themselves to an excellent examination question.

Think of the physiology of starvation as the body's metabolic adaptations to reduce protein breakdown.

Here are some definitions to avoid confusion (for more detail see Chapter 19, 'Carbohydrate Metabolism'):

Glucose is stored in the liver and muscles in the form of a multi-branched polysaccharide called glycogen. Glycogen is broken down by glycolysis to yield glucose-1-phosphate and glycogen.

Gluconeogenesis is the metabolic pathway that yields glucose from non-carbohydrate sources such as pyruvate, lactate, glycerol and amino acids.

What stores of energy does a 70 kg male possess?

Energy is stored as carbohydrate, protein and fat.

> 1600 kcal as glycogen
> 24 000 kcal in mobilisable protein
> 135 000 kcal in triacylglycerols

[kcal is an abbreviation for kilocalorie, which is equivalent to 1 large calorie (1c), or 1000 small calories (1000 c), or about 4.185 kJ (kilojoules)]

What are the 24-hour energy requirements of a 70 kg male at rest?

1600–2000 kcal per 24 hours (this may rise to 6000 kcal with stress).

If there is no energy intake, how does the body adapt?

Carbohydrate reserves (glycogen) only last approximately 24 hours, and less if the subject is exercising. Despite the exhaustion of glycogen, blood glucose levels are maintained. The brain cannot tolerate low blood glucose for even short periods and so the first priority of metabolism in starvation is to provide sufficient glucose to both the brain and red blood cells, both of which are absolutely dependent on this fuel source.

A lot of energy is stored in triacylglycerols; however, fatty acids cannot be converted into glucose to supply the brain or red cells because acetyl-CoA cannot be converted into pyruvate. The only other source of glucose available is amino acids derived from protein breakdown (i.e. muscle breakdown); however, survival depends on maintaining protein and muscle mass and, therefore, the second priority of metabolism in starvation is to preserve protein. Consequently, the body shifts its primary fuel source from glucose to fatty acids and ketones.

What adaptations occur during the first 24 hours of starvation?

As blood glucose levels begin to fall, insulin secretion is reduced and its counter-regulatory hormone, glucagon, is secreted, leading to mobilisation of triacylglycerols in fat and gluconeogenesis by the liver.

Concentrations of acetyl-CoA and citrate rise, which reduces glycolysis. Muscle uptake of glucose reduces secondary to the lack of insulin and, therefore, muscle also shifts to using fatty acid as fuel.

Pyruvate is no longer converted into acetyl-CoA and therefore pyruvate, lactate and alanine are exported to the liver for conversion into glucose.

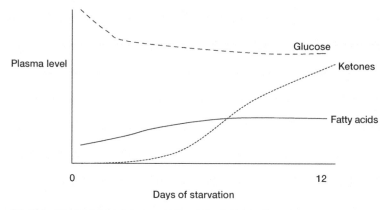

Fig. 20.1 Plasma glucose, ketone and fatty acid levels in starvation

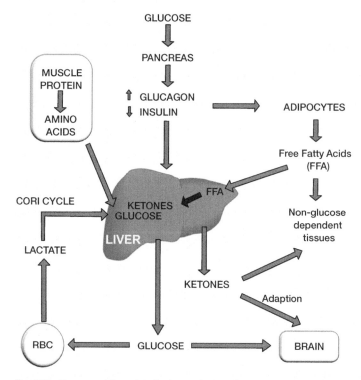

Fig. 20.2 Summary of the metabolic changes in starvation

What adaptations occur after 72 hours of starvation?

The most important metabolic change is the hepatic production of large amounts of ketone bodies (acetoacetate and 3-hydroxybutarate) from acetyl-CoA.

This occurs because gluconeogenesis depletes the supply of oxaloacetate, which is essential for acetyl-CoA to enter the Krebs cycle. Instead, the acetyl-CoA is used for ketogenesis.

The brain now begins to use acetoacetate (ketone body) for 30% of its energy requirements, i.e. adaptation has occurred.
The heart is also able to use ketones as an energy source.

What adaptations occur several weeks into starvation?

Ketones now become the major fuel source for the brain (>70%).
The effective conversion of fatty acids into ketones by the liver and their subsequent use by the brain markedly diminishes the need for glucose and, therefore, reduces muscle breakdown.

The duration of starvation compatible with life is determined by the size of the triacylglycerol stores.

Early starvation – reduction in energy expenditure, glycogen stores used within 24 hours, use of alternative fuels such as ketones to minimise protein wasting.

Late starvation – fatty acids, ketones and glycerol provide all of the energy requirements for the body, except for the brain and red blood cells, which still require a glucose source.

21. NAUSEA AND VOMITING

Nausea and vomiting are hazards of both general and regional anaesthesia. Post-operative nausea and vomiting (PONV) can be extremely distressing and some studies have found it to be as distressing as pain.

Define nausea and vomiting.

Nausea is the sensation of the need to vomit.
Vomiting is the involuntary, forceful expulsion of gastric contents via the mouth.

Describe the physiology of vomiting.

The physiology of vomiting is complex with multiple afferent and efferent pathways; an overview is helpful.

The chemoreceptor trigger zone (CTZ) lies in the floor of the fourth ventricle in the area postrema and is functionally outside of the blood–brain barrier. It contains dopamine (D_2) and serotonin ($5-HT_3$) receptors. The CTZ provides efferent input to the vomiting centre, which is located in the medulla. The vestibular system, peripheral pain pathways, intestinal chemoreceptors and the cerebral cortex all provide direct afferent input to the vomiting centre via cranial nerves VIII, IX and X.

Describe the process of vomiting.

Vomiting is an involuntary reflex and may be divided into two phases, a pre-ejection phase and ejection phase.

Pre-ejection phase:
• Nausea
• Sympathetic stimulation – tachycardia, tachypnoea, sweating
• Parasympathetic stimulation – salivation, upper and lower oesophageal sphincters relax, giant retrograde contraction of the small intestine.

Ejection phase:
• Respiration temporarily ceases mid-inspiration.
• Hyoid and larynx raise to open the crico-oesphageal sphincter.
• Glottis closes.
• Soft palate elevates to close off the nasopharynx.
• Contraction of the diaphragm and abdominal muscles results in a rise in intra-abdominal pressure.
• Gastro-oesophageal sphincter opens.
• Ejection of gastric contents.

What are the potential complications of vomiting?

Vomiting may result in potentially life-threatening complications:
• Aspiration (particularly if GCS is reduced)
• Wound dehiscence
• Electrolyte imbalance (loss of hydrogen, potassium and chloride)
• Dehydration
• Elevated intraocular and intracranial pressure.

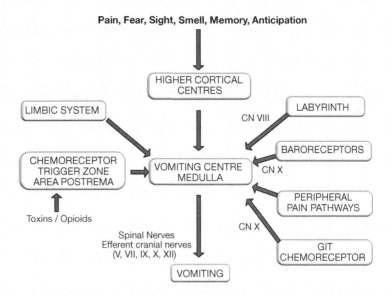

Fig. 21.1 Overview of nausea and vomiting

What are the main risk factors for PONV?

Divide the answer into patient, anaesthetic and surgical factors.

Patient factors
- Female gender
- Non-smoker
- Previous PONV
- History of motion sickness

Anaesthetic factors
- Use of N_2O
- Use of opiates
- Use of etomidate
- Use of neostigmine
- Hypotension

Surgical factors
- Middle ear surgery
- Ophthalmic surgery (especially squint-correction surgery)
- Gynaecology surgery

22. LIVER PHYSIOLOGY

The liver is a complex organ with multiple functions and as such plays a key role in homeostasis; its importance is best illustrated in acute liver failure.

There are a number of aspects of hepatic physiology that may be covered in an exam question and this answer should provide you with the pertinent key points.

Describe the anatomy of the liver.

- Adult liver weighs approximately 1800–2000 g.
- Divided into right and left hemi-liver plus caudate lobe.
- Histological unit of the liver is the lobule (*see* Fig. 22.1). Lobules are hexagonal in shape and have several portal triads located at their periphery.
- Portal triad is composed of hepatic artery, portal vein and bile duct.
- The central vein (branch of hepatic vein) is present in the centre of the lobule, surrounded by hepatocytes.
- Sinusoids traverse the lobule, draining blood from the peripheral portal triads to the central vein.
- Sinusoids also contain Kupffer cells, part of the reticuloendothelial system.
- Hepatocytes produce bile, which is excreted into the hepatic ducts of the portal triad via the bile canaliculi.
- Functional unit of the liver is the acinus (*see* Fig. 22.2), a diamond-shaped area of the liver supplied by a terminal branch of the portal vein and of the hepatic artery and drained by a terminal branch of the bile duct.

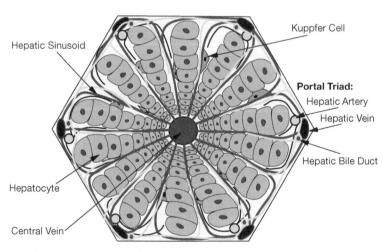

Fig. 22.1 Liver lobule

What are hepatic zones?

The liver acinus is divided into zones 1–3. The portal triad is composed of the hepatic artery, portal vein and bile duct. It is the portal triad that forms the centre of the acinus and, as such, forms zone 1. Blood becomes progressively poorer in oxygen and nutrients from zone 1 to zone 3 (i.e. zone 3 represents the microcirculatory periphery).

Zone 1 – Hepatocytes close to the portal triad. Surrounding blood is rich in oxygen and nutrients. Mitochondria-rich cells are present, which are suited to oxidative metabolism and glycogen synthesis.

Zone 3 – Hepatocytes at the periphery of the acinus, which receive blood that has already undergone exchange of gases and metabolites with cells in zones 1 and 2. Zone 3 is rich in smooth endoplasmic reticulum and cytochrome P450, making this the key region for drug and toxin biotransformation. It is also this zone that is most at risk of cellular damage during circulatory disturbances.

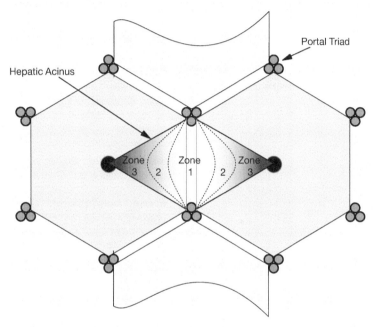

Fig. 22.2 Hepatic acinus

Describe the blood supply to the liver.

- The liver is an extremely vascular organ, receiving a blood supply of 100 mL/kg/min (approximately 1800 mL/min).
- It has a dual blood supply, receiving approximately 70% of its blood flow from the portal vein and 30% from the hepatic artery.
- The portal vein is formed by the union of the splenic vein and superior mesenteric vein and thus carries blood from the gastrointestinal tract to the liver.
- The hepatic artery is a branch of the coeliac artery.
- Hepatic portal vein blood only has an oxygen saturation of approximately 70%, and so it only provides around 40% of the liver's oxygen requirements.
- The hepatic artery provides approximately 60% of the liver's oxygen requirements.
- Normal hepatic oxygen extraction is less than 50%. However, this can increase in response to increased oxygen demand.

What factors affect blood flow to the liver?

- Blood flow through the hepatic artery is autoregulated (maintenance of constant flow despite changes in mean arterial pressure) down to a mean arterial pressure of approximately 60 mmHg. Below this, flow is pressure dependent.
- In contrast, blood flow through the portal vein is passive and dependent upon splanchnic blood flow.
- Therefore, only the arterial component of hepatic blood flow is controllable.
- The hepatic arterial blood flow is under intrinsic and extrinsic control.

Intrinsic control of hepatic arterial blood flow:
- **Myogenic response:** as the mean arterial pressure rises, the hepatic artery constricts to maintain a constant blood flow and vice versa.
- **Hepatic arterial buffer response** (arterio-venous reciprocity): as hepatic portal venous flow changes, the hepatic artery vasoconstricts or vasodilates reciprocally in order to maintain overall constant hepatic blood flow.

Extrinsic control of hepatic blood flow:
- **Sympathetic nervous system:** stimulation results in hepatic arterial vasoconstriction.
- **Drugs:** volatiles and noradrenaline reduce hepatic blood flow.
- **General anaesthesia and spinal anaesthesia:** both reduce hepatic blood flow.
- **Surgical handling of the liver:** reduces hepatic blood flow.

Classify and discuss the functions of the liver.

Think of a patient with hepatic failure, who may exhibit the following symptoms or signs because of loss of hepatic function: jaundice, encephalopathy, coagulopathy, ascites, raised intracranial pressure, hypoglycaemia, renal dysfunction, loss of vascular tone and immunosuppression.

Biotransformation: the liver plays a key role in the biotransformation of drugs, chemicals and toxins via the cytochrome P450 electron transport chain.
- **Phase 1 reactions** (Hydrolysis/Oxidation/Reduction):These provide a reactive group for subsequent phase 2 reactions. They generally reduce the activity of a drug but may sometimes produce a toxic or active intermediate. If the product is water-soluble following phase 1 reactions, it will not require further phase 2 reactions, but will be renally excreted.
- **Phase 2 reactions** (Glucuronidation/Acetylation/Sulphonation/Methylation): These involve conjugation of phase 1 products to increase water solubility allowing renal or biliary excretion of the compound.
- **Factors determining hepatic clearance:**
  o Proportion of unbound drug in the plasma (cf. highly protein-bound drugs)
  o Rate of drug presentation to the liver (i.e. flow limited) – important for drugs with high first-pass metabolism, e.g. morphine and lignocaine
  o Rate of enzymatic breakdown (i.e. capacity-limited) – important for drugs with low first-pass metabolism, e.g. diazepam and warfarin
  o May be increased or decreased by hepatic enzyme inducers or inhibitors respectively
  o Hepatic function, e.g. affected by disease processes such as cirrhosis

Synthetic function: synthesis of albumin, immunoglobulins, clotting factors (all except factor VIII), haptoglobin, C-reactive protein and anti-thrombin III.

Metabolic functions:
- **Carbohydrates** – the liver maintains blood glucose concentrations via glycogenesis, gluconeogenesis and glycogenolysis (*see* Chapter 19, 'Carbohydrate Metabolism' and Chapter 20, 'Starvation').
- **Proteins** – synthesises, transaminates or deaminates proteins. Converts ammonia into the less toxic urea.

- **Lipids** – synthesises cholesterol and triglycerides.
- **Ketone bodies** – produces acetoacetate and β-hydroxybutyrate.
- **Vitamins** – activates vitamin D.

Digestive functions: The liver produces bile. Bile is primarily used for the emulsification of dietary lipids to allow their absorption. In addition, bile is required for the absorption of fat-soluble vitamins A, D, E and K.

Storage functions:
- The liver stores approximately 100 g glycogen.
- Vitamins A, D, E, K.
- Copper.
- Iron (as ferritin).

Capacitance function: at any one time the liver can hold as much as 15% of the circulating volume and therefore can act as a large blood reservoir. Approximately half of this blood can be returned to the circulation during periods of sympathetic stimulation.

Immunological function: Kupffer cells form part of the reticuloendothelial system and have the function of removal of old erythrocytes, bacteria and other antigens via phagocytosis.

Give examples of some liver function tests.

Alanine and aspartate aminotransferases (ALT and AST)
- Released into the blood following hepatocelluar damage.
- Serum level does not correlate with extent of liver injury.
- ALT more liver-specific than AST.

Indicators of biliary tract disease
- Elevated conjugated bilirubin.
- Elevated alkaline phosphatase (ALP) and gamma-glutamyl transferase (GGT).

Indicators of hepatic synthetic function
- All clotting factors are synthesised by the liver except factor VIII.
- Prothrombin time (PT) indirectly determines the amount of available clotting factors and is therefore used to assess synthetic function.
- Serum albumin is difficult to interpret in the setting of critical illness because of renal and gastrointestinal losses; however, it will be reduced in chronic liver disease.

23. GASTRIC REGULATION

Describe what happens in the GI tract when a meal is anticipated.

There are three main phases of gastric regulation:

> Cephalic phase
> Gastric phase
> Intestinal phase.

Cephalic phase

These reflexes are decreased by stimulation of the sympathetic nervous system with, for example, pain, fear and anxiety.

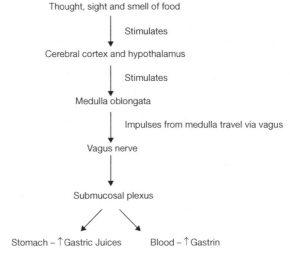

Thought, sight and smell of food

Stimulates

Cerebral cortex and hypothalamus

Stimulates

Medulla oblongata

Impulses from medulla travel via vagus

Vagus nerve

Submucosal plexus

Stomach – ↑Gastric Juices   Blood – ↑Gastrin

Fig. 23.1 Cephalic phase

Gastric phase

> As food and fluid enter the stomach, stretch and chemoreceptors are activated.
> This leads to a further increase in gastric secretions and increases peristalsis.
> The tone of the lower oesophageal sphincter is increased to prevent reflux of acid.
> Once the pH has reached 2, gastrin begins to exert a negative feedback to inhibit further acid secretion.

Intestinal phase

This begins when chyme (food mixed with gastric juices) enters the duodenum, causing the secretion of three main gut hormones:

> Gastric inhibitory peptide (GIP), which inhibits further gastric secretions and motility
> Secretin, which inhibits further gastric secretions
> Cholecystokinin (CCK), which inhibits stomach emptying.

Describe the function of these gut hormones.

There are four main hormones involved: gastrin, GIP, secretin and CCK.

Table 23.1 Functions of gut hormones

Hormone	Release stimulated by:	Actions
Gastrin	Cephalic phase Stomach distension Proteins in stomach ↑ pH of chyme in stomach	↑ Secretion of gastric juices ↑ Motility Encourages growth of mucosa Constricts LOS Relaxes pyloric and ileocaecal sphincters
GIP	Fatty acids in small intestine	↑ Insulin release Inhibits secretion of gastric juices Slows gastric emptying
Secretin	Acidic chyme in small intestine	Stimulates contraction of gallbladder to release bile Stimulates release of pancreatic enzymes Augments effect of CCK
CCK	Amino acids in small intestine Fatty acids in small intestine	Stimulates contraction of gallbladder to release bile Stimulates release of pancreatic enzymes Induces feeling of satiety Inhibits gastric emptying Enhances actions of secretin

Describe the sphincters present in the gastrointestinal tract.

A sphincter is a structure, usually made up of circular muscle, that surrounds the opening of a hollow organ or body and constricts to close it. Sphincters can be anatomical, where they are clearly different from the surrounding tissue, e.g. the anus, or functional where the histological distinction is not so clear, e.g. lower oesophageal sphincter. Sphincters can be under voluntary or involuntary control. There are many sphincters in the gastrointestinal tract:

> Upper oesophageal
> Lower oesophageal
> Pyloric
> Ileocaecal
> Sphincter of Oddi
> Anus

Upper oesophageal sphincter: This is at the level of the C5–6 vertebrae and is made up of the cricopharyngeal part of the inferior pharyngeal constrictor muscle. It is under conscious control and in its resting state it is usually constricted to avoid air being drawn into the stomach during breathing.

Lower oesophageal sphincter (also called the 'cardiac' sphincter): This is a functional sphincter, found at the junction between the non-keratinised squamous epithelium of the oesophagus and the simple columnar epithelium of the stomach. Its function is to prevent reflux of the acidic stomach contents into the oesophagus and so it is constricted at rest and has a pressure of 15–20 mmHg. The sphincter opens ahead of peristalsis during the process of swallowing to allow food and fluid to enter the stomach. It is supplied by the vagus nerve.

'Barrier pressure' describes the difference between LOS pressure and intragastric pressure. The closer the barrier pressure is to zero, the more likely it is that reflux will occur. So, reducing LOS tone or increasing intragastric pressure (e.g. pregnancy, full stomach, abdominal distension) makes reflux more likely.

Pyloric sphincter: This is an anatomical sphincter found at the junction of the stomach and duodenum. Its ring of muscle relaxes to allow chyme to pass out of the stomach. It is supplied by the coeliac ganglion.

Ileocaecal sphincter: An anatomical sphincter found at the junction of the small and large bowels. It prevents reflux of colonic material into the ileum.

Sphincter of Oddi: This is a ring of muscle that surrounds the bile and pancreatic ducts as they emerge into the lumen of the duodenum about halfway down its length. The sphincter controls the release of bile and pancreatic enzymes into the duodenum.

Anus: The gastrointestinal tract ends in a pouch called the rectum, where faeces are stored prior to defecation. At the exit of the rectum is the anorectal junction, a voluntary sphincter that is made up of an internal and an external ring of muscle. The internal anal sphincter is supplied by the hypogastric plexus. It is involuntary and will relax in response to stretching. The external anal sphincter is voluntary and supplied by the inferior rectal nerves.

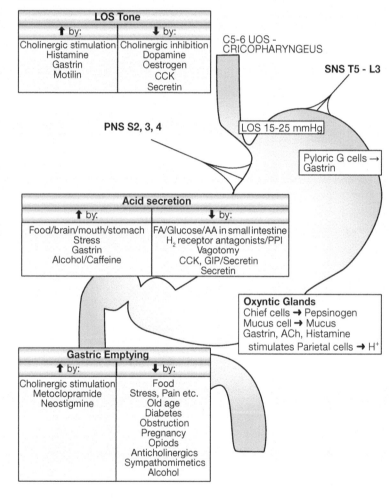

LOS Tone	
↑ by:	↓ by:
Cholinergic stimulation	Cholinergic inhibition
Histamine	Dopamine
Gastrin	Oestrogen
Motilin	CCK
	Secretin

C5-6 UOS - CRICOPHARYNGEUS

SNS T5 - L3

PNS S2, 3, 4

LOS 15-25 mmHg

Pyloric G cells → Gastrin

Acid secretion	
↑ by:	↓ by:
Food/brain/mouth/stomach	FA/Glucose/AA in small intestine
Stress	H_2 receptor antagonists/PPI
Gastrin	Vagotomy
Alcohol/Caffeine	CCK, GIP/Secretin
	Secretin

Oxyntic Glands
Chief cells → Pepsinogen
Mucus cell → Mucus
Gastrin, ACh, Histamine
stimulates Parietal cells → H^+

Gastric Emptying	
↑ by:	↓ by:
Cholinergic stimulation	Food
Metoclopramide	Stress, Pain etc.
Neostigmine	Old age
	Diabetes
	Obstruction
	Pregnancy
	Opiods
	Anticholinergics
	Sympathomimetics
	Alcohol

PNS	Parasympathetic nervous system
SNS	Sympathetic nervous system
UOS	Upper oesophageal sphincter
LOS	Lower oesophageal sphincter
FA	Fatty acids
AA	Amino acids
PPI	Proton pump inhibitors

Fig. 23.2 Overview of gastric regulation

24. TOTAL PARENTERAL NUTRITION

Questions on parenteral nutrition have appeared in the primary examination, albeit rarely, as the topic lends itself more towards the final examination. Nevertheless, as doctors who may be involved in prescribing total parenteral nutrition (TPN) within the critical care setting, examiners would expect a basic understanding of the indications, nutritional content requirements and complications associated with this form of feeding.

Parenteral nutrition is, by definition, administered intravenously. TPN supplies all daily nutritional requirements to the patient. In general, because TPN solutions are concentrated and therefore have the potential to cause venous thrombosis in peripheral veins, a central venous catheter is required.

What are the indications for TPN?

Where possible, the enteral route should always be used in preference to parenteral nutrition. However, where this is not possible, TPN should be considered.

> Anticipation of undernutrition (<50% of metabolic requirements achieved enterally) for >7 days.
> TPN may be indicated for severely undernourished patients unable to ingest large volumes of oral feed prior to surgery, radiation therapy or chemotherapy.
> Patients with disorders requiring complete gastrointestinal rest, e.g. ulcerative colitis/pancreatitis.
> Post-operative patients in whom enteral feeding has either not been possible or has failed after 5 days.

Describe the nutritional content of TPN.

TPN should be considered as a drug. Most hospitals in the UK now have a nutrition team comprising a physician, dietician and pharmacist, with the remit of reviewing patients with nutritional concerns and guiding safe use of parenteral nutrition.

Table 24.1 Basic adult requirements for TPN

Water	30–40 mL/kg/day
Energy	Medical patient 30 kcal/kg/day
	Post-operative patient 30–45 kcal/kg/day
	Hypercatabolic patient 45–60 kcal/kg/day
Amino acids	Medical patient 1 g/day
	Post-operative patient 2 g/day
	Hypercatabolic patient 3 g/day
Essential fatty acids	
Minerals	Acetate/Calcium/Chloride/Copper/Magnesium
	Potassium/Selenium/Sodium/Zinc
Vitamins	A/D/E/K/C/Folic acid/Thiamine/Pyridoxine/Niacin

Basic TPN solutions are prepared using sterile techniques. Solutions may be modified based on laboratory results (e.g. electrolyte disturbances), underlying disorders, hypermetabolism or other factors. Commercially available lipid emulsions are often added to supply essential fatty acids and triglycerides and 20–30% of total calories are usually supplied as lipids. However, withholding lipids and their calories may help obese patients mobilise endogenous fat stores and increase their insulin sensitivity.

Electrolytes can be added to meet the patient's needs. Patients who have renal insufficiency and are not receiving haemofiltration or who have hepatic failure require solutions with reduced protein content and a higher percentage of essential amino acids. For patients with respiratory failure, a lipid emulsion must provide most of the non-protein calories in order to minimise CO_2 generation.

How is TPN administered and monitored?

Ideally, TPN should be administered through a dedicated port of a central venous line. Strict asepsis must be used during administration. The infusion is started initially at 50% of the calculated requirements. Insulin may be required to maintain glycaemic control. Basic monitoring tests include daily weight, FBC, urea and electrolytes, and liver function tests.

What complications may occur with TPN?

With close monitoring by a nutrition team complication rates should be <5%, however complications related either to the central venous catheter (infection) or to the nutrition, may occur.

Volume overload – may occur when high daily energy needs require large volumes of fluid.

Glucose abnormalities – hyperglycaemia may occur (less commonly hypoglycaemia) and therefore regular blood glucose monitoring is essential.

Electrolyte disturbances – the most clinically important electrolytes to be monitored are sodium, potassium, magnesium and phosphate.

Metabolic bone disease – bone demineralisation develops in some patients receiving prolonged TPN (>3 months). The only remedy is to discontinue the TPN temporarily or permanently.

Hepatic complications – transient liver dysfunction on starting TPN is common, evidenced by increased hepatic transaminases, bilirubin and alkaline phosphatase. Delayed or persistent elevations may result from excessive quantities of amino acids. The pathogenesis of the hepatic complications is not known.

Gallbladder complications – include cholelithiasis and cholecystitis.

Refeeding syndrome – is a relatively rare but potentially fatal complication of TPN and a favoured examination question. The syndrome describes the severe hypophosphataemia and other metabolic complications that are seen in malnourished patients who receive concentrated calories via TPN. The syndrome was first described in Japanese prisoners of war after the Second World War.

Refeeding syndrome usually occurs within 72 hours of starting the feed. The syndrome results from a sudden shift from fat to carbohydrate metabolism with a sudden rise in insulin secretion leading to an increased cellular uptake of phosphate, potassium, magnesium and glucose. Serum levels of these electrolytes fall rapidly causing life-threatening systemic consequences including acute cardiac failure, confusion, coma, convulsions and even death. Prevention of the syndrome involves identifying patients at risk and introducing slow refeeding along with close monitoring and correction of electrolyte disturbances.

25. ACID–BASE BALANCE

A stable pH in body fluids is essential to maintain normal enzyme function, ion distribution and protein structure.

Homeostatic acid–base regulatory mechanisms aim to maintain a pH between 7.35 and 7.45 ([H+] of 45–35 nmol/L) via:

> *Buffers in tissue and blood*
> *Excretion of acids by kidneys and lungs*

Normal acid–base balance relies on the following variables:

> *pH ~ 7.40*
> *PCO_2 ~ 5.3 kP_a (40 mmHg)*
> *HCO_3^- ~ 24 mmol/L*

An acid–base disturbance occurs when at least two of these three variables are abnormal.

The primary change determines whether a disturbance is respiratory (alteration of PCO_2) or metabolic (alteration of the bicarbonate buffer system by means other than PCO_2).

Define the following:

Base: proton acceptor, or hydroxide (OH^-) producer, pH > 7.0

Acid: proton donor, pH < 7.0

The strength of an acid is defined by its ability to give up protons:
> **Strong acid** (e.g. HCl): fully dissociates in solution
> **Weak acid** (e.g. carbonic acid): does not fully dissociate, and together with its conjugate base, it acts as an acid–base buffer system to resist a change in pH.

pH: a measure of the acidity of a solution and is calculated as the negative logarithm to the base 10 of the hydrogen ion concentration.

> Normal serum pH is 7.40 (range 7.36–7.44).

pK_a: the pH of an acid at which it is 50% dissociated, or in equilibrium with its conjugate base. It is a measure of the strength of an acid (the lower the pK_a, the stronger the acid) and is calculated as the negative logarithm to the base 10 of the dissociation constant of an acid.

Acidosis: a process where there is acid accumulation or alkali loss.

Acidaemia: occurs when the arterial pH < 7.35 or [H^+] > 45 nmol/L.

Alkalosis: a process where there is acid loss or alkali accumulation.

Alkalaemia: occurs when the arterial pH > 7.45 or [H^+] < 35 nmol/L.

Standard bicarbonate: plasma concentration of bicarbonate when arterial PCO_2 has been corrected to 5.3 kP_a, haemoglobin is fully saturated and the body temperature is 37 °C. It represents what the actual bicarbonate would be after eliminating any respiratory component of acid–base disturbance.

Base excess (deficit): the amount of acid or base required to restore 1 litre of blood to normal pH at a $PaCO_2$ of 5.3 kP_a and at body temperature. It is negative in acidosis and positive in alkalosis, and is a useful marker of severity of the metabolic component of acid–base disturbances.

The **Siggaard–Anderson nomogram** can be used to derive the base deficit and standard bicarbonate if the pH, PCO_2 and haemoglobin are known.

What compensatory mechanisms exist?

These aim to restore the pH towards normal, and are based on maintaining the ratio $PaCO_2/[HCO_3^-]$; therefore, the variable in the compensatory response always changes in the same direction as the variable responsible for the primary imbalance.

Correction occurs when all three variables (pH, HCO_3^- and $PaCO_2$) are restored to normal levels.

> **Initial compensation is by intracellular buffering** (carbonic acid–bicarbonate buffer system and haemoglobin) and occurs within 2 hours.
> **Respiratory compensation** reaches its maximum by 24 hours and is by:
>   • **Hyperventilation** in the presence of a metabolic acidosis.
>   • **Hypoventilation** in the presence of a metabolic alkalosis.
> **Renal compensation** is by:
>   • **Increased acid (H^+) secretion and HCO_3^- retention** (reabsorption and regeneration) in the presence of a respiratory (and metabolic) acidosis.
>   • **Decreased acid (H^+) secretion and HCO_3^- retention** (reabsorption and regeneration) in the presence of a respiratory (and metabolic) alkalosis.

The generation of bicarbonate, through urinary excretion of ammonium and phosphate, restores the depleted HCO_3^- and buffer base reserves over 2–3 days.

Table 25.1 Primary changes and compensatory mechanisms in acid–base disorders

Primary disturbance	Initial imbalance	Compensatory response	Compensatory mechanism	Expected level of compensation
Metabolic acidosis	↓ HCO_3^-	↓ PCO_2	Hyperventilation	1.2 mmHg decrease in PCO_2 for each 1 mmol/L decrease in HCO_3^- (minimum PCO_2 of 1.3–1.9 kP_a in compensation)
Metabolic alkalosis	↑ HCO_3^-	↑ PCO_2	Hypoventilation	0.7 mmHg increase in PCO_2 for each 1 mmol/L increase in HCO_3^- (PCO_2 should not rise above 7–8 kP_a in compensation)
Respiratory acidosis	↑ PCO_2	↑ HCO_3^-		
• Acute			Intracellular buffering	1–2 mmol/L increase in HCO_3^- for every 10 mmHg increase in PCO_2
• Chronic			Renal: generation of bicarbonate via excretion of ammonium	3–4 mmol/L increase in HCO_3^- for every 10 mmHg increase in PCO_2
Respiratory alkalosis	↓ PCO_2	↓ HCO_3^-		
• Acute			Intracellular buffering	1–2 mmol/L decrease in HCO_3^- for every 10 mmHg decrease in PCO_2
• Chronic			Renal: decreased reabsorption of HCO_3^-, decreased excretion of ammonium	4–5 mmol/L decrease in HCO_3^- for every 10 mmHg decrease in PCO_2

Identify the abnormalities of these arterial blood gases: pH 7.0; PaCO$_2$ 7 kP$_a$; PaO$_2$ 7 kP$_a$.	Abnormality:	Acidaemia (pH < 7.4)
	Process:	Acidosis (excess production of acid, in the form of CO$_2$)
	Primary change:	Respiratory ($\uparrow$PaCO$_2$ and $\downarrow$PaO$_2$, i.e. type 2 respiratory failure)
	Acute v. chronic:	Likely acute as uncompensated
	Base excess/deficit:	Negative
	Standard bicarbonate:	Low in acute setting, as slow renal compensation is incomplete

What would you expect the pH to be in patients with a chronically elevated PaCO$_2$ at 7 kP$_a$?

In chronic respiratory acidosis, the renal compensatory mechanisms result in a chronic elevation of plasma bicarbonate, which in turn restores the pH to within the normal range. Typically, renal compensation is not complete, and the normal level of pH 7.40 is never reached.

How does metabolic compensation take place?

The increased PaCO$_2$ in the renal tubular cells results in an increased secretion of H$^+$ ions. Their secretion results in the following:

- Reabsorption of bicarbonate by the dissociation of carbonic acid
- Regeneration of bicarbonate by the excretion of H$^+$ with ammonia and phosphate in urine.

Metabolic compensation takes place over 2–3 days.

Describe the physiological process accounting for the low pH.

Respiratory acidosis is a consequence of hypoventilation or ventilation perfusion inequalities.

The resulting elevated PCO$_2$ disrupts the ratio of HCO$_3^-$ to PCO$_2$ and causes a drop in pH.

Comment on the PaO$_2$.

This is lower than normal, suggesting either a problem with ventilation, diffusion, shunt or a ventilation–perfusion mismatch. Assuming the inspired concentration of oxygen is known, the alveolar partial pressure of oxygen can be calculated using the alveolar gas equation. The A-a gradient can then be worked out and type of hypoxia can be assessed, to help establish the cause.

Define anion gap and list causes of an increased gap.

> The anion gap (AG) is the difference between measured cations (positively charged ions) and measured anions (negatively charged ions) in serum.
> This difference (gap) can be accounted for by the presence of unmeasured anions, such as albumin, lactic acid, ketones (β-hydroxybutyrate and acetoacetate), phosphates and sulphates.
> Classically it has been calculated using the equation:
> • AG = ([Na$^+$] + [K$^+$]) − ([Cl$^-$] + [HCO$_3^-$])
> • Normal range of 10–20 mmol/L
> • [K$^+$] may be excluded from the equation (as its value is negligible compared to the other measured ions) giving a normal AG range of 8–16 mmol/L.
> • Modern analysers now predict a normal range of 3–11 mmol/L.
> In the presence of acidic unmeasured anions, there is a secondary loss of bicarbonate ions due to their buffering capacity, but chloride concentration remains unchanged in order to maintain electroneutrality. The AG, therefore, becomes elevated.
> Clinically, it is useful in distinguishing the differential diagnosis of metabolic acidosis. A commonly used mnemonic to remember the causes of high AG metabolic acidosis is MUDPILES (**M**ethanol, **U**raemia, **D**iabetic ketoacidoasis (and ketoacidosis due to alcohol or starvation), **P**ropylene glycol, **I**ron/Isoniazid, **L**actic acidosis, **E**thylene glycol, **S**alicylates. A simpler one would be KULT (**K**etoacids, **U**raemia, **L**actic acids, **T**oxins).
> Note that in metabolic acidosis with a normal AG, there is usually a primary loss of bicarbonate ions (diarrhoea, renal tubular acidosis, Addison's disease), with a compensatory elevation in chloride concentration.

26. BUFFERS

What is the definition of a buffer?

An acid–base buffer solution resists a change of pH when an acid or base is added to it. It consists of a weak acid and its conjugate base (salt).

The general equation for a buffer system is:

HA (undissociated acid) $\leftrightarrow$ H⁺ (hydrogen ion) + A⁻ (conjugate base)

> **Le Chatelier's principle states that** if H⁺ ions are added to the solution, the equilibrium shifts to the left, and the H⁺ ions are 'neutralised' by the conjugate base, minimising an increase in free [H⁺] and maintaining a constant pH. If a base is added, H⁺ and OH⁻ react to form water, but more HA dissociates to maintain the [H⁺] constant, therefore the equation shifts to the right.

> By applying the Law of Mass Action, **(K_a = [H⁺] [A⁻]/[HA])**, the **Henderson–Hasselbach equation** can be derived and the (pK_a) for a buffer system can be calculated:

$$pH = pK_a + \log \text{[conjugate base]/[acid]}$$
$$\mathbf{pH = pK_a + \log [A^-]/[HA]}$$

(where **K_a** is the dissociation constant of a buffer and pK_a is the pH at which 50% of the buffer's acid is dissociated).

What is a buffer–titration curve?

> A titration curve is a plot of pH vs. the amount of acid or base added to a buffer solution (titration).
> It is useful for determining the pK_a of weak acids or bases.
> The pH is plotted on the y axis and the buffer composition on the x axis.

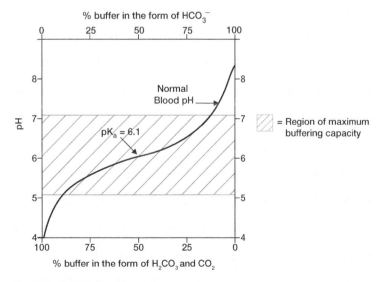

Fig. 26.1 Buffer titration curve

> For the bicarbonate and carbonic acid buffer system, on the left side of the plot, most of the buffer is in the form of carbon dioxide or carbonic acid and on the right side of the plot, most of the buffer is in the form of bicarbonate ion.
> The curve is sigmoid in shape, with greater pH changes occurring at the extremes of buffer compositions.
> If acid is added, the pH decreases, and the buffer shifts towards a greater H_2CO_3 and CO_2 concentration.
> Conversely, as base is added, the pH increases and the buffer shifts towards a greater HCO_3^- concentration.
> The flatter part of the slope represents the area of greatest buffering capacity where a shift in the relative concentrations of bicarbonate and carbon dioxide produces only a small change in the pH of the solution.
> The steeper part of the slope represents the area of least buffering capacity, where even a small shift in relative concentrations of acid and base produces a large change in the pH.
> At the central (equivalence) point, both acid and base are present in equal proportions, and the pH is equal to the pK_a (6.1) for the buffer.
> At the physiological blood pH of 7.4 (outside of the zone of greatest buffering capacity), small changes in the relative compositions cause a large pH change.
> Therefore, in order to maintain a constant pH, the body relies additionally on other buffer and organ systems.

What are the characteristics of an ideal buffer?

A good buffer solution must maintain a nearly constant pH when either acid or base is added. Two features render this possible:

> **Range of buffer** (defined as $pH = pK_a \pm 1$).
  • The buffer functions most effectively when its pK_a is within one unit of the desired pH of the solution.

> **Buffering capacity**
  • This is defined by the ratio of the concentrations of weak acid to conjugate base, which must remain fairly constant, such that the addition of acid or base will not cause a change of pH.

What are the physiological buffer systems in the body?

The bicarbonate/carbonic acid buffer system:
• This is the most important system.
• Despite it having a low pK_a (6.1) relative to blood pH, it is effective due to the ready excretion of carbonic acid in the form of CO_2 by the lungs, and the continuous regeneration of bicarbonate by the kidneys.
• It is more efficient at buffering acids since its efficiency increases as the pH falls.
• It is the main buffer system in the blood due to the abundance of plasma bicarbonate. The production of carbonic acid is catalysed by the enzyme carbonic anhydrase, which is present in red blood cells, but not in plasma.

The reaction for this buffer system is:

$$CO_2 + H_2O \leftrightarrow H_2CO_3 \leftrightarrow HCO_3^- + H^+$$

The Henderson–Hasselbalch equation for this buffer system is:

$$pH = 6.1 + \log [HCO_3^-] / [H_2CO_3]$$

and since H_2CO_3 is proportional to $PaCO_2$:

$$pH = 6.1 + \log [HCO_3^-] / 0.225 \times PaCO_2$$

(0.225 is the solubility coefficient for $PaCO_2$ in kP_a).

Haemoglobin:

- Acts as a blood buffer due to the imidazole groups of its histidine residues (each molecule has 38 histidine residues). Imidazole side chains are anionic and accept H^+.
- Deoxygenated haemoglobin (pK_a 8.2) dissociates more readily than oxygenated haemoglobin (pK_a 6.6), making it a better buffer and weaker acid (Haldane effect). The advantage at capillary level is that after O_2 has been offloaded, oxyhaemoglobin is reduced to deoxyhaemoglobin, which has a better buffering capacity, explaining why venous pH is only slightly more acidic than arterial pH.
- It has six times the buffering capacity of plasma proteins.

Plasma and proteins:

- These are effective buffers because both their carboxyl (COOH) and free amino (NH_2) groups dissociate. Intracellular proteins are equally important.

Phosphate:

- Plays a small role in the extracellular fluid, but is an important intracellular buffer due to its abundance and dissociation from phosphoric acid to dihydrogen phosphate and then to mono-hydrogen phosphate:

$$H_3PO_4 \leftrightarrow H_2PO_4^- + H^+ \leftrightarrow HPO_4^{2-} + H^+$$

Urinary buffering:

- Occurs in the proximal (PCT) and distal (DCT) tubules and collecting ducts.
- In the PCT, H^+ is secreted in exchange for Na^+ and combines with filtered HCO_3^- to form carbonic acid. This in turn dissociates into H_2O and CO_2, which move freely into the tubular cell. There, the reaction is reversed and the HCO_3^- formed enters the interstitium and later the plasma. Thus, for every H^+ secreted, one HCO_3^- is reabsorbed.
- Some phosphate buffering takes place in the PCT, but most of it occurs in the DCT and collecting ducts.
- H^+ combines with secreted NH_3 to form NH_4^+, which is excreted in the urine.
- Ammonia buffering takes place mainly in the PCT and DCT.
- Buffering by bicarbonate results in bicarbonate reabsorption, whereas buffering with phosphate and ammonia results in bicarbonate regeneration.

Table 26.1 List of physiological buffers

Body compartment	Buffer system	(pK_a)
Blood	Bicarbonate/carbonic acid	6.1
	Haemoglobin	7.8
	Plasma proteins	7.4
	Phosphate	6.8
Extracellular fluid	Bicarbonate/carbonic acid	
	Plasma proteins	
	Phosphate	
Intracellular fluid	Cellular proteins	
	Phosphate	
	Organic phosphates	
	Bicarbonate/carbonic acid	
Bone	Calcium carbonate	
Urine	Bicarbonate/carbonic acid	
	Phosphate ($HPO_4^- /H_2PO_4^{2-}$)	
	Ammonia (NH_3/NH_4^+)	9.0

What is the difference between 'open' and 'closed' buffer systems?

> **Closed buffers:** the total concentration of buffer within the cell is fixed, e.g. phosphate and haemoglobin. The addition of a strong acid or base results in maintenance of the pH, by shifting of the equation to the left or right, respectively. The buffering capacity is maximal when the pH = pK_a of the buffer system and is significantly reduced when the pH varies by more than 1 from the buffer's pK_a.

> **Open buffers:** the total concentration of buffer within a compartment is not fixed, e.g. bicarbonate/carbonic acid system. One of the components (H_2CO_3) is fixed while the other (HCO_3^-) varies inversely with the [H^+]. This is because CO_2 is highly permeable, therefore its intra- and extracellular concentrations are equal. As it is in equilibrium with H_2CO_3, it follows that the intracellular concentration of H_2CO_3 is fixed. The buffering capacity increases as the concentration of the non-fixed component (HCO_3^-) increases. Therefore intracellular pH increases, despite cell pH moving further away from the buffer's pK_a.

How much acid is produced by the body per day?

The body produces metabolic and respiratory acids. Metabolic acids are produced from metabolism of amino acids, phosphoproteins and phospholipids, and amount to 70 μmol/min or 0.1 mol/day.

Respiratory acids are formed from CO_2 production and amount to 200 mL/min or 8 mMol/min which equals 12 mol/day.

Other sources of acid production include:
- Lactic acid (strenuous exercise)
- Ketoacids (diabetes, alcohol, starvation)
- Failure of H^+ secretion by diseased kidneys (renal failure)
- Ingestion of acidifying salts (NH_4Cl and $CaCl_2$).

What effects does chronic renal failure have on acid–base balance?

> More acid is produced by metabolism than is excreted. This depletes extracellular buffers and reduces plasma bicarbonate levels.

> Reduced total number of functioning nephrons → reduced production and secretion of ammonia → reduced buffering of urinary H^+ → reduced tubular secretion of H^+.

> Excess K^+ causes intracellular alkalosis, which inhibits H^+ secretion.

> Bicarbonate reabsorption and regeneration are reduced.

> Excess acid may be buffered by calcium carbonate in bone, so contributing to renal osteodystrophy.

> Haemoglobin levels are reduced due to depressed production of new red blood cells from a diminished erythropoietin secretion.

> Plasma proteins may be diminished in the presence of increased glomerular permeability in certain conditions (glomerulonephritis/nephrotic syndrome).

27. RENAL BLOOD FLOW

The kidney receives 20–25% of cardiac output, i.e. 500–600 mL/min to each kidney.

More than 90% supplies the cortex via the renal artery, and less than 10% supplies the renal capsule and renal adipose tissue.

The cortex is supplied at 500 mL/min/100 g tissue. Some of this blood passes into the medulla, with perfusion rates of 100 mL/min/100 g tissue to the outer medulla and 20 mL/min/100 g tissue to the inner medulla.

> **HINT: REMEMBER THE RULE OF 5s**
> - *1/5 of cardiac output*
> - *500 mL/min to each kidney*
> - *500 mL/min/100 g tissue to the cortex*
> - *1/5 of this (100 mL/min/100 g tissue) to the outer medulla*
> - *1/5 of that (20 mL/min/100 g tissue) to the inner medulla*

Describe the anatomy of the kidney.

The renal artery enters each kidney at the hilum and divides into several branches. Interlobar arteries give rise to interlobular arteries that give rise to afferent arterioles, which supply the glomerular capillaries (site of filtration). Glomerular capillaries drain into efferent arterioles, which are portal vessels as they carry blood from one capillary network to another. In the outer two-thirds of the cortex, peritublar capillaries surround the proximal and distal convoluted tubules and collecting tubules. In the inner one-third of the cortex, the vasa recta surround the loops of Henle and collecting ducts.

What are the functions of renal blood flow (RBF)?

> - Provision of glucose and oxygen to meet the metabolic demands of renal tissue.
> - Removal of CO_2 and other products of metabolism.
> - Maintenance of GFR.
> - Provision of O_2 for active reabsorption of sodium.

Describe the autoregulation of renal blood flow.

Autoregulation describes the ability to maintain a constant RBF over a wide range of mean arterial pressures (MAP) or tissue perfusion pressures (PP) from 90–200 mmHg.

> - **Myogenic theory** – This is the most widely accepted explanation brought about by a direct contractile response of the afferent arteriolar smooth muscle to stretch. An increase in perfusion pressure results in smooth muscle contraction and an increase in the renal vascular resistance, so maintaining a constant blood flow.

> **Other factors affecting RBF include:**
> - Renal sympathetic nerve stimulation results in vasoconstriction of afferent arterioles thereby reducing RBF
> - Renal prostaglandins (PG) attenuate sympathetic-induced vasoconstriction through vasodilation, thereby increasing RBF
> - Angiotensin 2 vasoconstricts the efferent arterioles more than the afferent arterioles, thus maintaining glomerular filtration rate (GFR)
> - Tubuloglomerular feedback mechanism
> - Mediators present in blood vessel walls help to regulate GFR by vasodilatation (nitric oxide, NO) or vasoconstriction (endothelin).

Describe the tubuloglomerular feedback (TGF).

The rate of flow through the tubules feeds back (negatively) to affect glomerular filtration. The mechanism has three components:

> - Sensor: the macula densa in the distal tubular epithelium detects fluid delivery within the tubule
> - Transmission of signal to the glomerulus
> - Effector: vascular smooth muscle in the afferent arteriole adjusts GFR by vasodilatation or vasoconstriction.

As the fluid load in the tubule increases, the afferent arteriole vasoconstricts and GFR is reduced. The converse applies.

TGF is mediated by PG, thromboxane A_2, NO and endothelin, and plays a role in RBF autoregulation.

How can renal blood flow be measured?

RBF can be calculated by plasma clearance of para-aminohippuric acid (PAH), as a modification of the Fick principle.

> - **Fick principle:** Flow to an organ is equal to the uptake/excretion of a substance by an organ per unit time divided by the arterio-venous (A-V) concentration difference of that substance across that organ (L/min).
> - **Plasma clearance:** the volume of plasma cleared of a substance per unit time (mL/min). PAH, an organic acid is used because:
>   - it has a high extraction ratio (it is almost completely removed by the kidneys) via filtration and secretion, therefore its A-V concentration difference across the renal vascular bed is equal to the renal arteriolar concentration.
>   - it is neither utilised nor excreted by any other organ, therefore is peripheral venous plasma concentration is identical to its renal arterial concentration.
> - Applying the Fick equation, PAH uptake by the kidney is given by the product of urine PAH concentration and urine flow. The A-V concentration difference is substituted by peripheral venous plasma concentration as explained above. This gives us the equation for clearance.

Clearance of PAH = Urine [PAH] × urine flow/plasma [PAH]

> - Clearance helps us calculate renal plasma flow (RPF), since it is plasma, and not blood which is filtered.
> - RBF can then be deduced from RPF if the haematocrit (Hct) is known, by the equation: **RBF = RPF/1-Hct**.

28. GLOMERULAR FILTRATION RATE

What do you understand by the term glomerular filtration rate (GFR)?	Glomerular filtration rate is a unit of measure of kidney excretory function, and can be defined as the volume of plasma cleared of an ideal substance per unit time (or the volume of plasma filtered at the glomerulus per unit time).
	It is usually expressed as mL/min, and is approximately 125 mL/min or 180 L/day.
	Values in women are ±10% lower than those in men.
	The classification of chronic kidney disease is largely based on calculated or estimated GFR.
Define filtration fraction (FF).	This is the ratio of GFR to RPF (~0.16–0.2).
	Renal plasma flow (RPF) represents the total amount of potentially filterable fluid entering the kidneys (600–700 mL/min). Of this, 125 mL/min forms the GFR (20%) while the remainder continues into the efferent arterioles.
How can GFR be measured?	GFR can either be calculated (using the plasma clearance of a suitable substance, by applying the Fick principle) or estimated using prediction formulae (based on factors such as the patient's age, sex and serum creatinine level).

Estimated (eGFR)
The most commonly used are the Cockcroft and Gault (C&G) equation and formulas based on the modification of diet in renal disease study (MDRD).

- C&G: inaccurate in overweight individuals and in fluid overload.
- MDRD: most validated formula for eGFR and used in most laboratories. It does not require weight or height variables because results are reported normalised to 1.73 m^2 body surface area.

  Calculated applying the Fick principle and using the formula for clearance of a substance (inulin/creatinine):

$$\text{Clearance (GFR)} = \text{Urine concentration} \times \frac{\text{Urine flow}}{\text{Plasma concentration}}$$

How and why is inulin used to assess renal function?	Inulin, an exogenous polysaccharide with a molecular weight of 5200 Daltons, meets all the criteria of an ideal substance as follows:

- Freely filtered through the glomeruli (not bound to protein)
- Not reabsorbed nor secreted
- Not metabolised
- Not stored in the kidney
- No effect on the filtration rate
- Not toxic
- Easy to measure in plasma and urine.

The use of inulin is limited because of its expense and impracticalities.

Its administration requires a bolus followed by an infusion, and collection of blood and urine samples over several hours. Nowadays it is used mostly for research, where very accurate assessments of GFR are required.

Discuss alternatives along with their limitations.

Creatinine
> Urine [creat] may be elevated due to tubular secretion, but this is often cancelled out by plasma [creat], which is raised due to non-specific chromogens.
> In practice, creatinine clearance is no longer used to measure GFR, as a 24-hour urine collection is required, which is impractical for patients and leads to inaccuracies in measurement.
> It is affected by muscle mass, diet and tubular secretion. A trend in values, rather than a single measurement is more important when assessing renal function.
> It also remains within the normal range until a significant reduction in renal function occurs particularly in the elderly who have a reduced muscle mass.
> Drugs such as ACE inhibitors (ACEI) or angiotensin II receptor antagonists (ARB) may increase serum creatinine by up to 30%.

Urea
> Less reliable than creatinine because 40–50% of filtered urea may be reabsorbed by the tubules.
> Non-renal factors may affect serum levels (urea is raised with a high-protein diet, tissue breakdown, major gastrointestinal haemorrhage and corticosteroid therapy; lowered with a low protein diet and liver disease).

Cystatin C
> Endogenous substance, freely filtered but limited due to wide variation in serum levels.
> At present, it has no clinical role in GFR measurement.

What factors affect GFR?

These are the same as those governing filtration across any capillary bed:

> Permeability of capillaries
> Size of capillary bed (surface area)
> Hydrostatic and osmotic pressure gradients across the capillary wall (Starling's forces).

Capillary permeability
> Glomerular capillary wall is highly permeable due to its fenestrations.
> Neutral substances of < 4 nm diameter are freely filtered, but > 8 nm, their filtration approaches zero.
> Between 4 and 8 nm, their filtration is inversely proportional to diameter (Graham's law).
> The basement membrane's negative charge repels negatively charged ions, whose filtration is greatly reduced, e.g. albumin.
> The filtration of positively charged ions is slightly greater than that of neutral substances.

Size of capillary bed (surface area)
> Mesangial cells, located between the capillary endothelium and the basement membrane, have a contractile function, reducing the surface area available for filtration.
> Many vasoactive substances affect the mesangial cells, e.g. angiotensin 2 contracts while PGE2 relaxes.

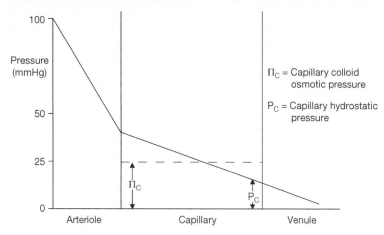

Fig. 28.1 Hydrostatic and osmotic pressures within a typical vascular bed

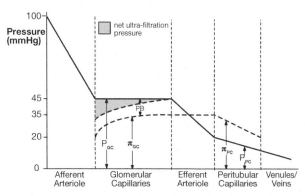

Fig. 28.2 Hydrostatic and colloid pressures within the renal vascular bed

Starling's forces

> The net filtration rate is a function of the forces favouring filtration and those opposing it, and can be described by the following equation:

$$GFR = K_f \, [(P_{GC} - P_B) - (\Pi_{GC} - \Pi_B)]$$

Where:
K_f = glomerular filtration coefficient (permeability $\times$ capillary bed surface area)
P_{GC} = hydrostatic pressure in glomerular capillary
P_B = hydrostatic pressure in Bowman's capsule
Π_{GC} = colloid osmotic pressure in glomerular capillary
Π_B = colloid osmotic pressure in Bowman's capsule

> P_{GC} is higher (45 mm Hg) than in other capillary beds (32 mm Hg) because:
  • Afferent arterioles are short and straight
  • Efferent arterioles have a relatively high resistance
> P_{GC} favours filtration and is opposed by:
  • Hydrostatic pressure in Bowman's capsule
  • Osmotic pressure gradient across the glomerular capillaries ($\Pi_{GC} - \Pi_B$)

- Π_B is usually negligible and the osmotic pressure gradient is generally equal to the pressure exerted by the plasma proteins within the glomerular capillaries (Π_{GC}).

The equation can therefore be expressed as:

$$GFR = K_f \, [P_{GC} - P_B - \Pi_{GC}]$$

- P_{GC} remains constant from afferent to efferent end of the glomerular capillary (45 mm Hg), as does the P_B (10 mm Hg).
- Π_{GC} rises from 20 mm Hg at the afferent end to 35 mm Hg at the efferent end because plasma proteins become progressively more concentrated as filtration occurs along the length of the capillaries.
- Just proximal to the efferent arteriole, the net ultrafiltration pressure is reduced to zero and filtration ceases.

Table 28.1 Starling pressures (mmHg) at the afferent and efferent arteriole

	Afferent end	Efferent end
P_{GC}	45	45
P_B	10	10
Π_{GC}	20	35
Net	**15**	**0**

29. RENAL HANDLING OF GLUCOSE, SODIUM AND INULIN

Using a straight line to represent the length of the proximal convoluted tubule (PCT), from the Bowman's capsule to the start of the loop of Henle, show the glucose, sodium and inulin concentrations. Explain the diagram and the physiology involved.

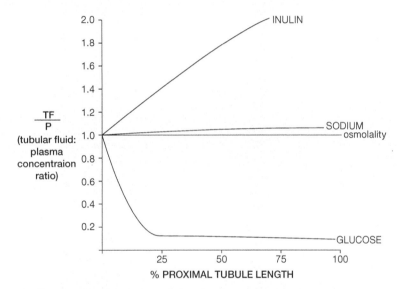

Fig. 29.1 Renal handling of glucose, inulin and sodium

> In health, glucose is completely reabsorbed so its concentration falls to zero along the length of the PCT (sharp decline in the first part of the PCT, with slower decline further down).
> Sodium is almost completely reabsorbed and is followed by passive diffusion of water, so its concentration remains unchanged (straight line).
> Inulin is filtered but not reabsorbed, so its concentration rises (sloped positive curve).

Table 29.1 Renal handling of various substances in filtrate per 24 hours

Substance	Filtered	Reabsorbed	Secreted	Excreted	Percentage reabsorbed	Location*
Na⁺ (meq)	26 000	25 850		150	99.4	P, L, D, C
K⁺ (meq)	600	560	50	90	93.3	P, L, D, C
Urea (mmol)	870	460		410	53.0	P, L, D, C
Creatinine (mmol)	12	1	1	12		P, L, D, C
Glucose (mmol)	800	800			100.0	P
Water (mL)	180 000	179 000		1000	99.4	P, L, D, C

*P = proximal tubules; L = loops of Henle; D = distal tubules; C = collecting ducts.

What are the transport mechanisms involved?

> **Passive diffusion** down chemical or electrical gradients, e.g. sodium ions from tubular lumen into tubular cell.
> **Facilitated diffusion** down chemical or electrical gradients:
> • Co-transport (symport) of glucose, amino acids, bicarbonate and other electrolytes with sodium
> • Antiport mechanism involving Na⁺ and H⁺ across the tubule wall.
> **Active transport** against chemical or electrical gradients, e.g. movement of sodium from tubular cell into the interstitium via the Na⁺-K⁺-ATPase pump.

The driving force behind the reabsorption of sodium and other ions is the Na⁺-K⁺-ATPase pump, which acts at the basilar wall of the tubular cell. It extrudes 3 Na⁺ into the interstitium in exchange for 2 K⁺ that are pumped into the cell. This creates a Na⁺ concentration gradient between the tubular lumen and cell such that sodium can diffuse passively into the cell from the lumen. The movement of other molecules and electrolytes is coupled to sodium reabsorption by antiport and symport mechanisms. Water diffuses along its concentration gradient. The K⁺ that is pumped into the cell passively diffuses out into the interstitium along its concentration gradient.

How much glucose is filtered by the kidney, and how much can be reabsorbed?

> 100% of plasma glucose is filtered.
> Active transport mechanisms become saturated at higher concentrations of solute and their maximum rate of transport (reabsorption) is reached. This is known as the transport maximum (T_m) for a given solute.
> Glucose reabsorption is proportional to the amount filtered, and hence to its plasma concentration multiplied by the GFR, up to the transport maximum, which is about 180 g/dL or 10 mmol/L of glucose in venous plasma.
> Once the renal threshold for glucose is reached, not all the filtered glucose is reabsorbed and glucose starts to appear in the urine.

What physiological factors increase the GFR?

These are the same factors that govern filtration across any capillary bed:

> Permeability of capillaries
> Size of capillary bed (surface area)
> Hydrostatic and osmotic pressure gradients across the capillary wall (Starling's forces).

The GFR is proportional to glomerular capillary pressure, which in turn depends on:

> Local autoregulation, mediated by renal sympathetic nerves
> Mean arterial pressure

30. FLUID COMPARTMENTS

Describe the major fluid compartments of the body in the adult.

> **Total body water** (TBW) varies depending on age, size, gender and fat content. It is approximately 60% of body weight (BW) in the average adult male (i.e. 42 L) and 50% in the average adult female. The remainder of the weight is made up of protein, minerals and fat. The main components of TBW are the extracellular and intracellular compartments.
> **Intracellular fluid** (ICF) makes up two-thirds of TBW (i.e. 28 L), and is contained within the phospholipid bilayer of the cell membrane.
> **Extracellular fluid** (ECF) makes up one-third of TBW (i.e. 14 L). This is divided into:
>   • **interstitial fluid** (ISF), which makes up 75% of the ECF (i.e. 9.5 L) and lies between cells, but outside the cell membrane
>   • **plasma**, making up 25% of the ECF (i.e. 3.5 L), contained within the vasculature
>   • **transcellular fluids** (TCF) (i.e.1 L), which are secreted fluids that are separated from the plasma by an epithelial layer (pleural, peritoneal, gastrointestinal fluids, CSF, intra-ocular fluids, sweat, saliva and bile), the so-called 'third space'
> **Total blood volume** (TBV) consists of plasma and red cell volume, and is 5–6 L.

Table 30.1 Fluid compartments for a 70 kg male

Compartment	% BW	% TBW	% ECF	Volume (L)
TBW	±60			42
ICF	40	67		28
ECF	20	33		14
• ISF	15	10.5	75	9.5
• plasma	5	3.5	25	3.5
• TCF	<1			1.0

Compare the adult with the neonate fluid compartments.

Table 30.2 Comparison of neonatal and adult fluid compartments

Compartment	Adult	Neonate
TBW (% BW)	60	75–85
Fat (% BW)	20–25	5–15
ECF (% BW)	20	30–45
ICF (% BW)	40	<40
Plasma (% BW)	5	5

Note that in premature babies, ECF exceeds ICF.

Describe the cell membrane and capillary barriers and the movement of molecules across them.

Cell membrane: this is a selectively permeable membrane that separates the intracellular contents from the extracellular environment. It consists of a phospholipid bilayer with hydrophobic heads on either side of the membrane and hydrophilic tails facing inwards. This arrangement allows fat-soluble molecules to diffuse easily across the membrane, but prevents the movement of polar molecules (amino acids, nucleic acids, carbohydrates, proteins and ions), which is enabled by transmembrane protein complexes such as pores, channels and gates. The movement of substances can be either 'passive' or 'active', i.e. with or without the expenditure of energy. The transport mechanisms involved include:

> **Passive osmosis and diffusion across a concentration gradient:** small molecules/ions such as CO_2 and O_2 can move across the plasma membrane by diffusion. The concentration gradient also sets up an osmotic flow for water.
> **Transmembrane protein channels and transporters:** molecules such as sugars, amino acids and certain products of metabolism may:
  • Passively diffuse through protein channels (such as aquaporins in the case of water) in facilitated diffusion, or
  • Actively be pumped across the membrane by transmembrane transporters.
> **Endocytosis:** cell membrane creates a vesicle, capturing the substance and internalising it, e.g. phagocytosis. This is a form of active transport.
> **Exocytosis:** the membrane of a vesicle fuses with the plasma membrane, expelling its contents into the extracellular environment, e.g. hormones and enzymes.

Capillary wall: consists of a single layer of simple squamous epithelium and a basement membrane (basal lamina). Capillaries connect arteries and veins within organ systems across a branched network called the capillary bed. The more metabolically active an organ is, the larger the capillary bed. Small molecules (<3 nm) such as water, oxygen and carbon dioxide cross the capillary wall through the space between cells (paracellular transport), while larger molecules (>3 nm) such as albumin and other large proteins pass through transcellular transport carried inside vesicles. There are three main types of capillaries:

> **Continuous:** uninterrupted lining with tight junctions and complete basal lamina. Allow passive diffusion of lipid-soluble molecules and movement of small molecules such as water and ions through intercellular clefts. Skeletal muscle and skin have numerous transport vesicles, whereas CNS (blood–brain barrier) has few, so sealing the paracellular space.
> **Fenestrated:** endothelial cells have pores or windows (60–80 nm in diameter) and a complete basal lamina. Allow a limited amount of proteins to diffuse. They are located in intestines, pancreas, endocrine glands and renal glomeruli.
> **Sinusoidal:** large open-pore (30–40 μm in diameter) capillaries, large gaps between cell junctions and a discontinuous basal lamina. Allow red and white blood cells (7.5–25 μm diameter) and serum proteins to pass. Present in bone marrow, lymph nodes, liver, spleen and adrenal glands.

How are the body compartment volumes estimated?

Dilutional techniques are used to estimate compartment volumes. An indicator dye is injected into the compartment to be measured. The dye should distribute throughout that compartment, but remain contained within it. The concentration of the dye is measured and the mass administered is known. Thus, using the formula for volume of distribution (V_d = mass of dye/ concentration), the compartment volume can be estimated.

Some compartments are derived (ICF, ISF and TBV).

Table 30.3   Methods of measurement of fluid compartments

Compartment	Characteristic of indicator	Indicator
TBW	Freely diffusible substance	Deuterium oxide Antipyrine
ECF	Substances that do not enter cells	Inulin Thiocyanate Thiosulphate
ICF	*TBW – ECF*	
Plasma	Substances confined to plasma	Radiolabelled albumin Evan's blue dye
Red cell volume		Radiolabelled red cells
TBV	*Plasma volume × 100/(100 – haematocrit)*	
Interstitial fluid	*ECF – plasma volume*	

What factors regulate body water?

Water balance governs the ICF, and sodium balance regulates the ECF compartments. (mnemonic WISE: **W**ater regulates **I**ntracellular; **S**odium regulates **E**xtracellular)

The control of TBW is linked to the secretion of antidiuretic hormone (ADH/vasopressin) by the posterior pituitary.

ADH is secreted in response to:

> Hyperosmolarity (threshold 1–2%) detected by osmoreceptors in the hypothalamus, outside the blood–brain barrier. Similarly, osmoreceptors stimulate thirst
> Volume depletion (ECF) detected by low-pressure baroreceptors in great veins, atria and pulmonary vessels, and high-pressure baroreceptors in the carotid sinus and aortic arch (threshold 7% change in volume)
> Angiotensin II (AGII)
> Other: pain, exercise, stress, emotion, nausea and vomiting, standing, nicotine, morphine, barbiturates, carbamazepine.

ADH secretion is reduced in response to:

> Low osmolarity
> Increased ECF volume
> Alcohol

The renal effects of ADH on water balance include:

> Increased water permeability in cortical collecting tubule (V2 receptors)
> Increased water and urea permeability in medullary collecting tubule
> Increased retention of water
> Reduced urine volume

Other ADH effects include:

> Release of factor 8 by the endothelium (V2)
> Platelet aggregation and degranulation (V1)
> Arteriolar vasoconstriction (V1)

Sodium balance governs the ECF volume (as water passively diffuses across membranes when sodium is reabsorbed) and is regulated by:

> Dietary sodium intake
> ECF volume (baroreceptors) and ADH secretion
> GFR and tubuloglomerular feedback.
> Renin–angiotensin–aldosterone system:
  • Efferent arteriolar vasoconstriction to maintain GFR
  • Direct sodium reabsorption
  • Secretion of aldosterone from adrenal cortex
  • Increased ADH
  • Increased thirst (water retention)
  • Negative feedback on renin release

> Aldosterone and other adrenocortical hormones:
>   • Reabsorption of NaCl (30–90 minute latent period)
>   • Excretion of K^+
>   • Secretion of H^+
>   • Accompanied by changes in ADH.
> Rate of tubular secretion of K^+ and H^+
> Atrial natriuretic peptide (ANP) and other natriuretic hormones:
>   • Secreted by atrial myocytes in response to atrial stretch due ECF expansion (from high NaCl intake or IV infusion of saline)
>   • Actions include natriuresis (by an increase in GFR and tubular excretion of sodium), reduction in BP (by reduced responsiveness of vascular smooth muscle to vasoconstrictors) and reduced secretion of aldosterone, ADH, renin and consequently AGII.

What is the effect of a sudden IV infusion of 5% dextrose?

> 5% dextrose is a hypotonic solution and therefore gets distributed equally throughout all the fluid compartments. It can be thought of as water because the dextrose gets metabolised leaving behind water, which diffuses freely.
> Intravascular volume will thus increase only minimally (by approximately 70 mL if 1 L was administered).
> This is less than the 7–10% threshold needed to stimulate the baroreceptors.
> However, the plasma osmolarity will decrease enough to stimulate the osmoreceptors (1–2% threshold) and therefore ADH secretion will decrease, increasing renal water excretion.

What is the effect of an IV infusion of 1 L 0.9% saline solution?

This is an isotonic solution and results in ECF expansion, diuresis and natriuresis as explained below:

> Sodium will diffuse from areas of high concentration to those of lower concentrations and will be followed by water
> The cell membrane is impermeable to sodium and thus the distribution of the saline (water) administered will be confined to the ECF with 75% (750 mL) in the ISF and 25% (250 mL) in the plasma
> The plasma expansion from 3.5 to 3.75 L is enough (7% increase) to be detected by the baroreceptors and ADH secretion is reduced
> The increased sodium load and ECF expansion will cause an increase in ANP secretion and natriuresis, and inhibition of the renin–angiotensin–aldosterone system.

31. OSMOREGULATION

Define the following terms:	**Osmosis:** the diffusion of water molecules (solvent) across a semi-permeable membrane, from a dilute solution to a concentrated solution.
	Osmotic pressure: the pressure required to prevent solvent migration by osmosis across a semi-permeable membrane. Applying pressure to the more concentrated solution can prevent the movement of water to the region of greater solute concentration.
	Osmole: reflects the concentration of osmotically active particles in solution.
	1 osmole = amount of solute that exerts an osmotic pressure of 1 atm when placed in 22.4 L of solution at 0 °C.
	For substances that do not dissociate, e.g. glucose, 1 osmole = 1 mole.
	For substances that dissociate into two osmotically active particles, e.g. NaCl, 1 osmole = 1 mole/2 (i.e. 1 mole = 2 osmoles).
	Osmolarity: the number of osmoles (or mosmoles) of solute in 1 L of solution, osm/L. As it is temperature dependent, it poses a potential source of inaccuracy.
	Osmolality: the number of osmoles (or mosmoles) in 1 kg of water (pure solvent), osm/kg. It is not influenced by temperature and is therefore more accurate than osmolarity.
How do you calculate plasma osmolality?	A simple formula, which sums up the major solutes, may be used:

$(2 \times Na^+)$ + glucose + urea

This adds up to approximately 290 mosmol/kg H_2O.

What are the colligative properties of water?	These are properties of solutions that depend on the number of solute particles, but not on their nature, i.e. they depend on the osmolarity of a solution:

> Lowering of vapour pressure
> Elevation of boiling point
> Depression of freezing point
> Osmotic pressure.

How do you calculate osmotic pressure?	Dilute solutions behave in a similar way to ideal gases, i.e. osmotic pressure (P) is related to temperature (T) and volume (V) in the same way that an ideal gas is.

Applying the van't Hoff equation: **PV = nRT**

Where:
n = number of particles and **R** = universal gas constant (n/V = osmolality), we can calculate the value of osmotic pressure of plasma as follows:

$$P = nRT/V$$
$$= 290 \text{ mosm/kg } H_2O \times 8.32 \text{ J/K} \times 307 \text{ K}$$
$$= 740\,729.6\,P_a$$
$$= 740.7\,kP_a$$
$$= 7.33\,atm\,(5629.3\,mmHg)$$

How do you measure osmotic pressure?

Osmometers capable of detecting temperature changes of 0.002 °C are used. They utilise one or more of the colligative properties of water:

> 1 mole of a solute added to 1 kg of water will depress the freezing point by 1.86 °C (e.g. grit salt on the icy roads causes the ice to melt).
> The molar concentration of a solute causes a directly proportional reduction in vapour pressure (Raoult's law).

What is oncotic pressure (colloid osmotic pressure)?

Electrolytes account for more than 99% of plasma osmolality and osmotic pressure. Plasma proteins contribute to the remaining <1%, which is the colloid osmotic (oncotic) pressure, and amount to 25–28 mmHg. Despite its small number, oncotic pressure is significant, as it is the major determinant of retention of fluid within the capillaries.

What are the body's osmoreceptors?

These are cells of the anterior hypothalamus, located outside the blood–brain barrier. They respond to changes in osmolality and stimulate thirst and the secretion of vasopressin.

What are the actions of vasopressin (antidiuretic hormone, ADH)?

ADH stimulates V2 receptors on collecting ducts, which increases adenylate cyclase activity. This causes fusion of pre-formed water channels on the apical membrane resulting in increased permeability of the collecting ducts to water. Other ADH effects include:

> Stimulates thirst
> Release of factor VIII by the endothelium
> Platelet aggregation and degranulation
> Arteriolar vasoconstriction
> Glycogenolysis in the liver
> Brain neurotransmitter
> Secretion of ACTH from the anterior pituitary gland.

What stimulates water intake?

Multiple factors are involved in regulating water intake.

> An increase in plasma osmolality (with effective increase in osmotic pressure) stimulates osmoreceptors in the anterior hypothalamus, which in turn control thirst and simulate us to drink. ADH release also stimulates thirst.
> Extracellular fluid (ECF) volume depletion stimulates the renin–angiotensin system. The resultant increase in circulating angiotensin II acts on a specialised receptor in the diencephalon concerned with thirst. Baroreceptors appear to be involved as well when ECF volume is low.
> Dryness of the pharyngeal mucous membranes causes the sensation of thirst.
> Psychological and social factors also play a role.

32. ACTION POTENTIALS

Questions about nerve action potentials (AP) are fairly common. Consider starting off by drawing a diagram of an AP. Remember to be accurate with the values of your membrane potentials.

Can you describe the action potential travelling along a mixed nerve?

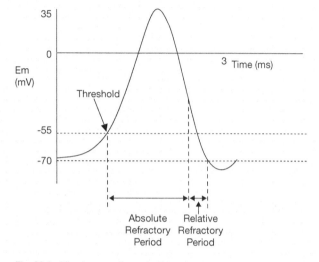

Fig. 32.1 Mixed nerve action potential

The term *action potential* describes the depolarisation above threshold potential, and subsequent repolarisation of a nerve axon resulting in the propagation of a nerve impulse along that axon. The easiest way to describe this is in a series of steps relating to the diagram of the AP:

> The inside of each cell in the body is negative relative to its surroundings. The potential difference across the cell membrane is called the membrane potential (E_m) and is governed by the membrane's relative permeability to sodium (Na^+) and potassium (K^+) ions. When the cell is at rest, it is relatively more permeable to K^+ than Na^+ and so the resting membrane potential approaches the equilibrium potential of K^+. In a mixed nerve this E_m is -70 mV.

> Nerve, muscle cells and pacemaker cells are able to generate APs. When a stimulus causes a movement of charge across the membrane, there is a movement away from the resting membrane potential. If the inside of the cell becomes more positive, this is called depolarisation whereas if it becomes more negative, this is referred to as hyperpolarisation. Depolarisation in a nerve cell is caused by the movement of Na^+ ions into the cell.

> If a nerve cell becomes depolarised, e.g. by distortion opening Na^+ channels in the mechanoreceptors of the skin, the movement of the membrane potential towards zero causes opening of voltage-gated Na^+ channels. Once a Na^+ channel opens, it will close again automatically after a millisecond or so. Therefore, if the initial stimulus is not strong enough to cause enough Na^+ channels to open to allow enough Na^+ into the cell to bring the E_m to threshold potential, the membrane potential will fall away from zero and become more negative as the K^+ equilibrium is re-established. Consequently, no AP will be generated.

> If, however, the initial stimulus is strong enough, enough channels will open to allow an influx of Na^+ that will raise the membrane potential to the threshold level of $-55\,mV$. If this level is reached, then a positive feedback effect occurs on the Na^+ channels, causing large numbers of them to open. Consequently, there is an explosive influx of Na^+ raising the membrane potential above 0 to $+35\,mV$. So, the AP is an 'all-or-nothing' event – the membrane either reaches threshold level or does not.

> These Na^+ channels opened by positive feedback will still close rapidly, as before. As the membrane potential nears the equilibrium potential of Na^+ ($+70\,mV$), the diffusion of Na^+ ions into the cell slows. The maximum membrane potential is defined by the relationship of the Na^+/K^+ equilibrium and, therefore, the size of the AP is fixed, and not dependent on the size of the stimulus. Similarly, the duration is fixed, because this is dependent on the length of time that the Na^+ channels remain open, and this time is fixed.

> Once the Na^+ channels close, repolarisation occurs by the movement of K^+ ions out of the cell to restore the resting membrane potential. This happens as voltage-gated K^+ channels open in the face of an AP, allowing the movement of the K^+ out of the cell along its diffusion gradient. These K^+ channels remain open after the Na^+ ones have closed, therefore allowing the resting membrane potential to be re-established. This process is called delayed rectification. Following only a few APs, the net change in number of Na^+ and K^+ ions in and outside the cell is small. However, after many APs, the changes become significant and the balance across the membrane is restored using the Na^+-K^+ pumps.

> An inactivated Na^+ channel cannot reopen until it has returned to near resting membrane potential. This explains the absolute refractory period that follows each AP, where the nerve cell cannot be excited, no matter how large the stimulus. The relative refractory period follows the absolute refractory period, and here, another AP can be generated with a supra-maximal stimulus.

How does the AP move along the axon of a nerve?

In an unmyelinated axon the AP moves rather like a wave; local currents spreading in front of the AP cause a change in membrane potential and bring the membrane to threshold potential to spark the propagation of the AP. The AP can only flow in one direction as the axon behind it will be refractory.

Myelin acts as insulation because the charge cannot leak from the axon in an area covered by the myelin, and so charge density is maintained. In the 'nodes of Ranvier', i.e. the spaces between the myelinated areas, the charge can escape; the net effect is that the AP jumps from node to node. This is called saltatory conduction. So, the myelin increases the AP's velocity, and its insulating effect allows axons to be of smaller diameter (without myelination, conduction is fastest in axons with larger diameters).

What is the Gibbs–Donnan equilibrium?

'Diffusion of permeable ions across a semipermeable membrane down their concentration gradient is balanced by the electrostatic attraction of impermeable ions (e.g. proteins) trapped on the inside of the membrane'.

What is the Nernst equation?

The Nernst equation calculates the electrical potential for an individual ion, thus helping to predict how each ion affects the cell membrane potential. It represents the electrical potential required to balance a given ionic concentration gradient across a membrane so that there is no net flux.

$$E_m = \frac{RT}{ZF} \times \ln \frac{[ion]^{OUT}}{[ion]^{IN}}$$

Where:

$[ion]^{OUT}$	Extracellular concentration of that ion (in moles/cubic metre)
$[ion]^{IN}$	Intracellular concentration of that ion (in moles/cubic metre)
E_m	Membrane equilibrium potential
R	Universal gas constant
T	Absolute temperature
Z	Valency
F	Faraday's constant

Because R, T and F are constants and Z is 1 for the majority of ions in which we are interested, the Nernst equation can be simplified to:

$$E_m = 61.5 \times \log_{10} \frac{[ion]^{OUT}}{[ion]^{IN}}$$

What is the Goldman constant field equation?

This calculates the value of the overall membrane potential taking into account the permeabilities and concentration gradients of each ion.

$$V_m = \frac{RT}{F} \ln \left(P_{Na^+} \frac{[Na^+]^{OUT}}{[Na^+]^{IN}} + \frac{P_K [K^+]^{OUT}}{[K^+]^{IN}} + \frac{P_{Cl}[Cl^-]^{OUT}}{[Cl^-]^{IN}} \right)$$

Where:

V_m = Membrane potential
R = The permeability of that ion (in meters/second)

33. CEREBRAL BLOOD FLOW

Cerebral function is dependent upon cerebral blood flow (CBF) and oxygenation. An understanding of the physiology of CBF regulation is essential in order to manage patients who may have decompensated intracranial pathology or injuries.

Basic concepts

> Global CBF: 50 mL/100 g brain tissue/minute.
> White matter blood flow: 20 mL/100 g/minute.
> Grey matter blood flow: 70 mL/100 g/minute.
> Resting oxygen consumption of the brain: 50 mL/minute (20% of total body oxygen requirements).
> Regional CBF varies depending on metabolic rates of local areas of brain.
> CBF exhibits autoregulation – the maintenance of constant blood flow despite changes in cerebral perfusion pressure (CPP).
> CPP = mean arterial pressure (MAP) – [Intracranial Pressure (ICP) + CVP]. N.B. CVP is often omitted from this equation.
> Normal CPP is approximately 70–80 mmHg.
> Cerebral blood flow: myogenic theory vs. local metabolites.
> CBF is autoregulated between an MAP range of 50 and 150 mmHg (curve is shifted to the right in hypertensive patients).

Myogenic theory of cerebral autoregulation.

A change in perfusion pressure results in a myogenic response in the cerebral vascular smooth muscle in order to maintain constant CBF. For example, a hypertensive response during exercise with an increase in MAP results in cerebral vasoconstriction thus keeping CBF constant. Conversely, a fall in MAP will result in cerebral vascular smooth muscle relaxation causing vasodilatation thus maintaining CBF.

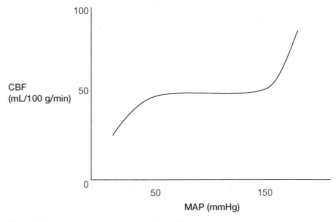

Fig. 33.1 Autoregulation of cerebral blood flow

Metabolic theory of cerebral blood flow.

CBF and cerebral metabolism are coupled. Thus, regional CBF varies with metabolic activity. Products of metabolism (H^+/K^+/adenosine/nitric oxide) cause vasodilatation. Thus, CBF matches metabolic requirements.

What are the effects of changes in PaO_2 and $PaCO_2$ on CBF?

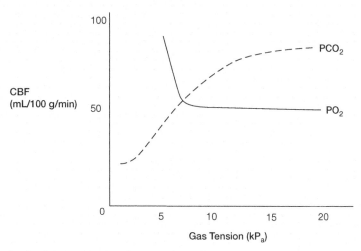

Fig. 33.2 Physiological control of cerebral blood flow

CBF increases linearly between a $PaCO_2$ range of 3 and 10 kP_a. Outside this range CO_2 reactivity is lost. This has clinical implications: hypocapnia can result in intense cerebral vasoconstriction and ischaemia; hypercapnia can result in increased intracranial blood volume, which may result in a rise in ICP.

CBF increases below a PaO_2 of 8 kP_a due to hypoxic vasodilatation. Clinical implication: in patients with head injuries hypoxia may lead to further rises in ICP and result in brain ischaemia.

Do anaesthetic drugs have any effect on CBF?

> **Volatiles:** all increase CBF and reduce Cerebral metabolic oxygen requirements ($CMRO_2$), thus uncoupling CBF from $CMRO_2$.
> **N_2O:** increases CBF and increases $CMRO_2$.
> **NMBA:** do not affect CBF.
> **Induction drugs:** With the exception of ketamine, all other induction agents reduce $CMRO_2$, CBF and ICP. Ketamine increases ICP.

How does temperature affect CBF?

Cerebral metabolic requirement for oxygen ($CMRO_2$) falls by 7% per 1 °C decrease in core body temperature. As a result, CBF parallels this reduction in $CMRO_2$.

What effect does brain injury have on cerebral blood flow?

Brain injury can lead to loss of cerebral autoregulation in injury-affected areas of the brain, resulting in the development of a pressure-dependent perfusion area. Thus, a fall in CPP may lead to secondary ischaemic brain injury.

What is the Monro–Kellie doctrine?

The skull is a rigid box containing brain tissue (80%), blood (12%) and CSF (8%). The volume of the box is constant, so an increase in volume of any one of the intracranial constituents must be accompanied by a parallel reduction in the volume of another constituent if ICP is to remain constant.

What is the normal ICP?

> 10–15 mmHg – normal.
> Above 20 mmHg – elevated ICP.

What are the common causes of raised ICP?

> **CSF** – hydrocephalus.
> **Brain** – tumours/oedema/contusions.
> **Blood** – haematoma/cerebral aneurysm.

Draw a graph to show how ICP is related to intracranial volume (ICV).

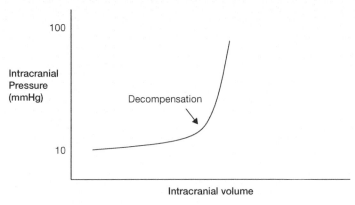

Fig. 33.3   Effect of intracranial volume on intracranial pressure

As intracranial volume increases (e.g. cerebral oedema secondary to a traumatic brain injury) there is no initial rise in ICP as compensatory mechanisms occur such as a reduction in intracranial venous blood volume and an increase in CSF absorption combined with CSF movement into the spinal compartment. When these mechanisms are exhausted any further small increase in intracranial volume results in a large increase in ICP, i.e. decompensation has occurred.

What is the vasodilatory cascade?

In head-injured patients, the vasodilatory cascade describes the vicious cycle that develops if there is a reduction in cerebral perfusion pressure. Conversely, the vasoconstriction cascade describes the treatment of the above situation.

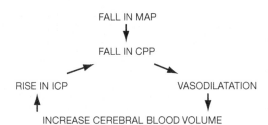

Fig. 33.4   Vasodilatory cascade

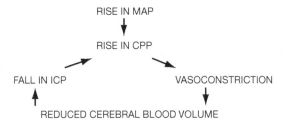

Fig. 33.5   Vasoconstriction cascade

Describe the physiological management of the head-injured patient.

Applying the above physiological principles, the following goals are aimed for when managing patients with head injuries:

ABC approach

Maintain oxygenation: Keep PaO_2 >10 kP_a as hypoxia will cause cellular ischaemia and raise ICP through vasodilatation

Maintain CPP >70–80 mmHg to ensure adequate CBF and to prevent the vasodilatory cascade **(CPP = MAP – ICP)**. The ICP in an unconscious patient can be presumed to be >20 mmHg; therefore, MAP should be maintained at around 90 mmHg. This may require fluids and/or vasopressors. Ensure good venous drainage of the head by positioning the patient at 30° head up tilt, do not obstruct venous drainage with endotracheal tube ties but use tape instead to secure the ETT. Ideally, ICP should be monitored, but this is monitoring usually available in specialist centres only.

Reduce ICP: Maintain normocapnia and normoxia. Hypercapnia and hypoxia will both increase cerebral blood volume and, therefore, ICP, according to the Monroe–Kellie doctrine.

- Sedate adequately and paralyse the patient to avoid straining.
- Consider the use of furosemide (0.25–1.0 mg/kg) or mannitol (0.25–1.0 g/kg) or hypertonic saline to decrease ICP by reducing cerebral oedema.

Reduce CMRO$_2$: Consider infusions of propofol or midazolam to reduce cerebral metabolism, or in certain situations thiopentone to induce a 'thiopentone coma'.

- Treat pyrexia.
- Therapeutic hypothermia: CMRO$_2$ decreases by 7% for every 1 °C fall in temperature and is paralleled by a fall in CBF. This may help to control ICP but cooling has not been shown to improve outcomes in head-injured patients.
- **Prevent/treat seizures** that cause a dramatic increase in CMRO$_2$.
- Maintain **normoglycaemia**.

Do not administer hypotonic fluids such as 5% dextrose, which will increase brain oedema as they cross the disrupted blood–brain barrier.

34. CEREBROSPINAL FLUID

What is CSF?

> Cerebrospinal fluid (CSF) is the clear colourless fluid that bathes the brain and spinal cord acting as a fluid layer for protection of the central nervous system (CNS).

Where is CSF produced?

> CSF is produced by the four choroid plexuses located in the third, fourth and lateral ventricles.
> Produced at a rate of approximately 0.3 mL per minute.
> Total volume of CSF is approximately 150 mL, which equates to approximately 10% of intracranial volume.
> 450 mL of CSF is produced per day and so CSF volume is replaced three times every 24 hours.
> CSF is derived from plasma filtration and subsequent secretion by the choroid plexuses.
> CSF is one of the three determinants of intracranial pressure (the other two being brain tissue and blood volume).
> In situations of raised intracranial pressure, CSF production remains relatively constant; however, CSF absorption increases thereby reducing total CSF volume (see Chapter 33, 'Cerebral blood flow').

Describe the circulation of CSF.

> CSF flows from the lateral ventricles through the foramen of Monro into the third ventricle and from there via the aqueduct of Sylvius into the fourth ventricle.
> CSF leaves the ventricular system via the midline foramen of Magendie and lateral foramen of Lushka, entering the subarachnoid space of the brain and spinal cord.
> CSF is absorbed into the dural venous sinuses via arachnoid villi and granulations that project into the dural sinuses.

What is the relevance of the blood–brain barrier (BBB)?

> Plasma constituents do not pass freely into the CSF. This phenomenon is known as the BBB.
> Anatomical and physiological factors involved in maintaining the BBB are:
>   • Tight junctions and fenestrated choroidal capillaries within the brain
>   • Specialised bidirectional transport system for ions, glucose and amino acids.

Describe the normal CSF composition.

Reference values for CSF are as follows:

Protein	0.15–0.45 g/L
Osmolality	280–300 mmol/L
Sodium	135–145 mmol/L
Potassium	2.6–3.0 mmol/L
Chloride	115–125 mmol/L
Calcium	1.00–1.40 mmol/L
Magnesium	1.2–1.5 mmol/L
Lactate	1.1–2.4 mmol/L
pH	7.28–7.40
Creatinine	50–110 µmol/L
Glucose	2.8–4.4 mmol/L
Urea	3.0–6.5 mmol/L

A comparison of the composition of CSF and plasma reveals that:

> CSF proteins are ~1% that of plasma, resulting in reduced buffering capability
> CSF calcium levels are ~50% that of plasma
> CSF glucose levels are ~60% that of plasma
> CSF chloride and magnesium levels are higher than plasma.

What investigations can be performed on a CSF sample?

Important information about CSF can be derived from the following parameters:

> Opening pressure: traditionally measured in cm H_2O (normal = 10–15 lying down, 20–30 sitting up). Elevated in raised intracranial pressure
> Macroscopic appearance, e.g. xanthochromia
> Total and differential cell count
> Bacterial culture and sensitivity
> Protein and glucose
> Analysis of immunoglobulins (detect chronic CNS inflammatory conditions)
> Cytology.

What changes in CSF cell counts occur with CNS infection?

CSF normally contains a small number of cells (usually lymphocytes and monocytes) and the total cell count is less than 5 cells/mm³. An increase in cell counts suggests either an infection of the CNS or a number of pathological CNS conditions. The differential cell count provides further information regarding the possible cause of the CNS disease.

> **Increased neutrophils** may indicate bacterial meningitis. Other causes of an increased neutrophil count include a cerebral abscess, seizures and CNS haemorrhage.
> **Increased lymphocytes** may indicate viral meningitis. Lymphocyte counts are also elevated in meningitis due to TB, syphilis, and fungal and parasitic infections. Degenerative diseases of the CNS, such as multiple sclerosis, will also generate elevated lymphocyte counts.
> **'Mixed reaction'**, an increase in neutrophils, lymphocytes and plasma cells. This is characteristic of TB meningitis, fungal meningitis and chronic bacterial meningitis.
> **Increase in plasma cells** is a feature of TB meningitis.
> **Leukaemic cells** indicate meningeal infiltration by haematological malignancy.

Can biochemical analysis of CSF be diagnostic?

> **CSF total protein:** The CSF normally contains less than 0.45 g/L protein. Increased levels may be found in:
> * Infection
> * Blood contamination
> * Chronic inflammatory disorders of the CNS (TB, syphilis, Guillain–Barré)

> **CSF electrophoresis:** Electrophoretic separation of CSF proteins and detection of CSF immunoglobulin.
> CSF immunoglobulin can arise from three causes:
> * Secondary to an increase in plasma immunoglobulin, e.g. multiple myeloma
> * Impairment of the blood–brain barrier
> * Local synthesis in the CNS, e.g. in multiple sclerosis the increase in CSF immunoglobulin is characterised by an oligoclonal pattern of immunoglobulin synthesis and this can be detected in 90% of patients with MS.

> **CSF glucose:** Low levels of CSF glucose suggest:
> * Infection (local metabolism by white cells)
> * Hypoglycaemia (although CSF glucose is of limited diagnostic utility and the plasma glucose concentration must be known in order to interpret the CSF glucose level properly).

> **Polymerase chain reaction (PCR)** is a technique to rapidly amplify a defined region of DNA or RNA. PCR has been used to detect the presence of bacterial pathogens (e.g. syphilis and TB) and viral pathogens (e.g. HIV) in the CSF.

35. AUTONOMIC NERVOUS SYSTEM

Many anaesthetic agents and neuroaxial blocks interfere with the autonomic nervous system (ANS). However, there are occasions when we seek to manipulate the autonomic system deliberately, using various drugs (e.g. inotropes, β-blockers) and manoeuvres (e.g. valsalva). This question has a wide scope and can lead onto a variety of topics including the vagus nerve, autonomic reflexes and drugs acting on the autonomic system.

What is the autonomic nervous system?

The ANS is a collection of nerves and ganglia that are involved in the involuntary control of homeostasis and the stress response.

Describe the structure of the autonomic nervous system.

> The ANS consists of two divisions, the parasympathetic nervous system (PNS) and the sympathetic nervous system (SNS). The PNS is involved in 'Rest and Digest' processes (picture Mr Parasympathetic sitting on the toilet, sphincters open and reading a newspaper with eyes accommodated). The SNS is involved in 'Fight-or-Flight' processes (just imagine what you are going to feel like at the exam – dilated pupils, sweaty, tachycardic, tachypnoeaic, dry mouth and shivering!).

> The ANS receives afferent information from chemoreceptors, baroreceptors, mechanoreceptors and from regions within the central nervous system. Once processed, it relays this information through efferent pathways to target tissues (e.g. cardiac muscle, smooth muscle and glands).

> The efferent pathways of the PNS and SNS consist of a pre-ganglionic fibre, an autonomic ganglion and a post-ganglionic fibre. (N.B. The exception to this is the SNS innervation of the adrenal gland where there is only a single pre-ganglionic fibre that terminates on the adrenal medulla. The adrenal medulla then acts like a glorified 'post-ganglionic' fibre and releases neurotransmitters/hormones into the bloodstream.)

Pre-ganglionic fibres (myelinated type B fibres):

> The cell bodies of the PNS pre-ganglionic fibres lie within the nuclei of III, VII, IX and X cranial nerves and also in the lateral grey horns of the second to fourth sacral segments. These fibres are long and form the craniosacral outflow tract.

> The cell bodies of the SNS pre-ganglionic fibres lie within the lateral grey horns of the first to twelfth thoracic segments and the first to third lumbar segments. These fibres are short and form the thoraco-lumbar outflow tract.

Autonomic ganglia:

> The PNS ganglia are known as terminal ganglia as they are located close to or within the wall of the target tissue.

> The SNS consists of two types of ganglia: the paravertebral ganglia (also called the sympathetic trunk) and the prevertebral ganglia. The paravertebral ganglia lie on either side of the vertebral column from the base of the skull to the coccyx. The prevertebral ganglia (e.g. coeliac, superior mesenteric and inferior mesenteric ganglia) lie anterior to the vertebral column next to the major arteries.
> White rami communicantes connect SNS pre-ganglionic fibres to paravertebral ganglia.

Post-ganglionic fibres (unmyelinated type C fibres):
> PNS post-ganglionic fibres are short and their cell bodies lie within the autonomic ganglia.
> SNS post-ganglionic fibres are long and their cell bodies lie within the autonomic ganglia.
> Grey rami communicantes connect SNS ganglia to spinal nerves.

Neurotransmitters:
> All PNS and SNS pre-ganglion fibres are cholinergic (they release acetylcholine).
> Whereas all PNS post-ganglionic fibres are also cholinergic, only those SNS post-ganglionic fibres innervating sweat glands are cholinergic.
> All other SNS post-ganglionic fibres are adrenergic (they release noradrenaline).
> The adrenal medulla, which acts like a 'glorified' SNS post-ganglionic fibre, releases adrenaline (80%) and noradrenaline (20%).

Receptors:
> Receptors sited within all autonomic ganglia and on the adrenal medulla are nicotinic acetylcholine receptors (nAChR).
> Receptors on the effector organs innervated by the PNS are muscarinic acetylcholine receptors (mAChR) while those innervated by the SNS are adrenergic receptors (either α or β).
> Muscarinic acetylcholine receptors are also located on sweat glands that are innervated by the SNS.

Which organs are not under dual innervation from the ANS?

Most target tissues receive dual innervation from the ANS. However, structures that only receive SNS innervation are the sweat glands, arrector pili muscles, adipose cells, kidneys and most blood vessels. The lacrimal glands only receive PNS innervation.

Compare and contrast the PNS and SNS.

Table 35.1 Comparison of the PNS and SNS

Function	Rest and digest	Fight or flight
Pre-ganglionic fibres	Craniosacral tract	Thoracolumbar tract
	Long	Short
	Cholinergic	Cholinergic
Ganglia	Terminal	Paravertebral or prevertebral
	nAChR	nAChR
Post-ganglionic fibres	Short	Long
	Cholinergic	Adrenergic
Target tissues	Dual innervation to most target tissues except lacrimal glands	Dual innervation to most target tissues except sweat glands, arrector pili muscles, adipose cells, kidney and most blood vessels
	mAChR	α and β receptors

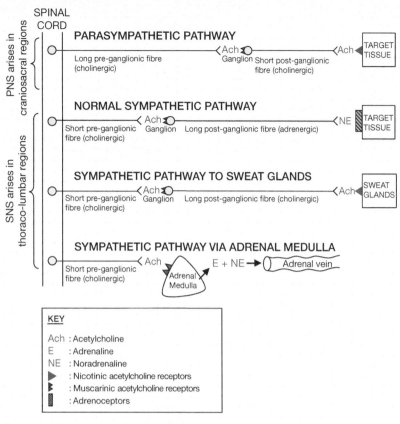

Fig. 35.1 Schematic representation of the ANS

36. CHILD VERSUS ADULT

This is a relatively straightforward question, but to answer it well you must structure your answer as there is a considerable amount of information to get across in a short space of time. Be systematic.

Describe the physiological and anatomical differences between a neonate and an adult.

In comparison to adults, children differ in the following anatomical and physiological ways:

Respiratory system:
> Relatively larger head, short neck, large tongue and narrow nasal passages.
> High anterior larynx (level C2/3 compared to C5/6 in the adult).
> Large U-shaped floppy epiglottis.
> Narrowest point of the larynx is at the level of the cricoid cartilage (in adults it is at the laryngeal inlet).
> Trauma to the small airway can easily lead to oedema and airway obstruction. 1 mm oedema can narrow an infant's airway by 60% (resistance $\propto 1/radius$).
> Equal angles of mainstem bronchi (in adults the right main bronchus is more vertical).
> Obligate nasal breathers.
> Compliant chest wall with horizontal ribs.
> Diaphragmatic breathing > intercostal breathing.
> Diaphragmatic movement restricted by relatively large liver.
> Relatively fixed tidal volume. Increase in minute ventilation achieved by increasing respiratory rate.
> Higher alveolar ventilation 100–150 mL/kg/min compared with 60 mL/kg/min in adult.
> Born with only 10% of the total number of alveoli as adults. Alveoli develop over first 8 years.
> Closing volume is larger than FRC until 6–8 years of age resulting in airway closure at end-expiration. Consider use of IPPV and PEEP.
> Sinusoidal respiratory pattern, no end-expiratory pause (inspiratory/expiratory ratio 1:1).
> Higher basal oxygen consumption 6 mL/kg/min compared with 3.5 mL/kg/min in the adult.
> Higher risk of apnoea.
> As a result of all of the above points, hypoxaemia occurs more rapidly.

Cardiovascular system:
> Circulating blood volume 85 mL/kg compared with 70 mL/kg in adult.
> Neonatal myocardium consists of more non-contractile connective tissue.
> Stroke volume is relatively fixed.
> Cardiac output is therefore largely rate dependent and neonates tolerate bradycardia poorly.
> Cardiac output 200 mL/kg/min.
> Parasympathetic nervous system better developed than sympathetic, meaning bradycardia occurs frequently with hypoxia or vagal stimulation.
> Asystole is the most common form of cardiac arrest and ventricular fibrillation is uncommon.
> Transitional circulation may revert to fetal circulation if neonate becomes hypoxic, acidotic, hypercapnic or hypothermic.
> Haemoglobin higher in neonate: 16–20 g/dL.
> Right ventricular mass equal to left ventricular mass until 6 months of age, resulting in right axis deviation on the ECG.

Central nervous system:
> Myelination is incomplete in the first year of life.
> Skull non-rigid with open fontanelles.
> MAC infant > neonate > adult.
> More sensitive to opiate-induced respiratory depression and apnoea.
> Immature neuromuscular junction that is very sensitive to non-depolarising muscle relaxants but relatively resistant to suxamethonium (use 1.5 mg/kg).
> Spinal cord ends at L3 (L1 by age 2 years).

Renal system:
> Higher total body water (80%) at birth.
> Increased extracelluar fluid (ECF) resulting in higher volumes of distribution of drugs.
> Renal immaturity resulting in poor handling of water excess or excess sodium.
> Poor renal hydrogen ion excretion.
> Glucose reabsorption is limited.
> Glomerular filtration and tubular reabsorption reduced until 6–8 months of age.
> Renal blood flow is 6% of cardiac output at birth rising to 18% of cardiac output at 1 month (compared with 20% in adult).
> GFR at term is 30 mL/min increasing to 110 mL/min by age 2 years.

Liver:
> Immature liver has fewer selective pathways to metabolise drugs.
> Low hepatic glycogen stores means hypoglycaemia occurs readily with prolonged fasting.

Temperature homeostasis:
> Poor temperature regulation in neonates.
> Large body surface area/volume ratio.
> High heat loss.
> Higher thermoneutral temperature (temperature below which an individual is unable to maintain core body temperature) 32 °C for a term infant compared with 28 °C for an adult.
> Infants <3 months of age cannot shiver.
> Utilise non-shivering brown fat thermogenesis.

37. PREGNANCY

This question is best answered by considering each system in turn. The list below is not exhaustive, but should certainly be enough to pass.

Can you describe the physiological changes associated with pregnancy?

Haematology:
> **Plasma volume increases:** this increases preload and V_D of polar drugs. It increases by 50% by term.
> **RBC mass increases:** but plasma increases more than RBC, causing physiological anaemia.
> **WBC increase:** to 12×10^9/L by term, with a further increase to 30×10^9/L during labour.
> **Platelets reduce:** due to consumption.
> **Albumin decreases:** this increases the free active proportion of plasma-bound drugs.
> **Plasma oncotic pressure reduces:** increases the risk of oedema.
> **Plasma cholinesterase reduces:** the effect of suxamethonium is offset by the increased V_D.
> **Hypercoagulable:** all clotting factors increase except XI and XIII. BT, PT and APTT shortened. High risk of thromboembolic complications.
> **CRP and ESR increase.**

Cardiovascular system:
> **Stroke volume and heart rate increase:** cardiac output increases by up to 60% by term (8 L/min).
> **Systemic vascular resistance reduces:** reduction in DBP > SBP leading to an increased pulse pressure. This is due to oestrogen and progesterone. Maintenance of SVR is governed by sympathetic drive, which is diminished by central neuroaxial blockade.
> **Left ventricular mass increases:** ECG shows left axis deviation, ST depression and even a flat or inverted T-wave. Systolic murmur almost universal at term, but note that a diastolic murmur is not normal.
> **Vena caval compression:** reduces venous return and preload, decreased cardiac output, decreased BP and engorged verterbral veins.
> **Aortic compression:** occurs from 20 weeks gestation. Increases afterload, decreases cardiac output and utero-placental blood flow. This is decreased by avoiding supine position and using at least 15° lateral tilt.

Respiratory system:
> **Anatomy:** capillary enlargement and mucosal congestion can lead to voice changes and difficulty breathing in some women. The diaphragm is elevated by 4 cm, thoracic circumference increases as the ribs 'splay' out and breathing becomes largely diaphragmatic by term.
> **Volumes:** FRC reduces by up to 20% and closing volume encroaches on FRC, leading to airway closure and increasing the risk of hypoxia. This is made worse when supine, obese or multiple pregnancy. VT increases but TLC and VC remains unchanged.

> **Ventilation:** respiratory rate and minute ventilation increase. Dead space increases due to bronchodilation.
> **Mechanics:** chest wall compliance reduces but lung compliance remains unchanged.
> **Oxygen consumption increases:** by up to 60%, increasing the risk of developing hypoxia during induction of anaesthesia.
> **ABG:** pH increases (to ~7.5), PO_2 increases (to ~14 kP$_a$), PCO_2 reduces due to hyperventilation (to ~3.5 kP$_a$) and HCO_3^- reduces (to ~18 mmol/L).

Gastrointestinal system:
> **Barrier pressure reduces:** due to increased intragastric pressure.
> **Gastric emptying is reduced:** this occurs during labour due to the effects of pain and opiates.
> **Risk of aspiration increases:** this returns to normal levels 48 hours post partum.

Renal:
> **Renal blood flow and GFR increase:** by up to 50%. Urea and creatinine levels reduce, meaning that a 'normal' creative level in pregnancy is abnormal.
> **Glycosuria and proteinuria:** common.

Central nervous system:
> **Epidural space reduces:** due to the engorged extradural venous plexus. CSF volume is also reduced. Hence reduced volumes of local anaesthetic agents are required during central neuroaxial blockade (reduce dose by one-third). There is also an increased risk of inadvertent intravascular catheter placement.
> **Anaesthesia:** MAC decreased. Inhalational induction faster (as raised MV more significant factor that raised CO in this case). Following labour, woman has reduced strength in respiratory muscles for around 4 hours. Anaesthesia compounds this effect and reduces ability to cough.

Endocrine:
> **Thyroid:** increases in T3 and T4, may suppress TSH.
> **Insulin:** increased secretion from hypertrophied beta cells, but increased production of 'anti-insulin' hormones, e.g. cortisol. Gestational diabetes can result. Glucose crosses placenta by facilitated diffusion to protect fetus from fluctuating maternal levels.

38. PLACENTAL TRANSFER

What are the main functions of the placenta?

> Gas exchange
> Nutrient and waste exchange
> Transfer of immune complexes
> Hormone synthesis, e.g. HCG, oestrogens, progesterone, TSH, prostaglandins.

Describe the mechanisms by which substances are transferred across the placenta.

Placental transfer is subject to exactly the same rules governing transfer of substances across all semi-permeable phospholipid membranes. Mechanisms of transfer include:

> **Simple diffusion**, e.g. O_2 and CO_2
> **Facilitated transport**, e.g. glucose
> **Secondary active transport**, e.g. amino acids
> **Active transport**, e.g. iron and calcium
> **Pinocytosis**, e.g. IgG
> **Bulk transport.**

What factors affect the transfer of substances across the placenta?

All substances present in the maternal circulation are potentially available to the fetus. The following factors govern transfer across the placenta.

> **Lipid solubility:** The more lipid-soluble a substance is, the more readily it will diffuse across a lipid membrane, and so the placenta.
> **Degree of ionisation:** The more ionised a substance is, the less easily it diffuses across the placenta.
> **Degree of protein binding:** Only the unbound ('free') substance is available to cross any membrane, and so a highly bound substance will not cross the placenta readily. Pregnant women have relatively lower total protein contents of their blood and so theoretically a higher free fraction of a given substance might be present.
> **pH:** This affects the degree of ionisation of the drug, as dictated by its pK_a. Also, acidosis decreases protein binding.
> **Molecular weight:** Substances with a molecular weight <600 Daltons cross readily.
> **Concentration gradient across the placenta:** This affects speed of transfer.

Local anaesthetics are often used during labour. Describe the transfer of local anaesthetics from the mother to the fetus.

> Bupivacaine is the most commonly used local anaesthetic, given either as epidural or subarachnoid injection. It is used because it has fewer motor effects than other drugs available and has a relatively long duration of action.
> It can cross the placenta, but less readily than lignocaine because its pK_a is higher than lignocaine's, making it more ionised at physiological pH.
> The fetus has a lower pH than its mother, and so there is a risk of 'ion trapping', where the drug crosses into the fetus, becomes more ionised, and therefore cannot move out again. This effect is exacerbated if the fetus becomes more acidotic, risking local anaesthetic toxicity.

Describe the transfer of pethidine.

> Pethidine is the most commonly used opioid for labour pain and can be prescribed by the midwives in most UK maternity units.
> It is a highly lipid-soluble drug and so it passes freely across the placenta reaching equilibrium in about 6 minutes and reaching maximum levels in the fetus at around 2–3 hours.
> It is metabolised to norpethidine, which is less lipid soluble and therefore remains in the fetus much longer.
> Norpethidine has little analgesic value and causes sedation and respiratory depression and is pro-convulsant. Its half-life in the mother is up to around 20 hours, but in the neonate can be as much as 62 hours.

Describe the Bohr effect in relation to placental gas exchange.

Consider drawing the oxyhaemoglobin dissociation curve and using it to illustrate your answer.

> The Bohr effect describes the movement to the left or right of the oxyhaemoglobin dissociation curve, depending on the surrounding CO_2 tension and the resulting pH.
> Ambient CO_2 diffuses into red blood cells and dissociates to form $H^+ + HCO_3^-$. This causes the curve to shift to the right, as there is a reduction in the affinity of haemoglobin for oxygen. This encourages offloading of oxygen to the tissues.
> This mechanism is important in the utero-placental circulation. As the mother's blood flows through the uterus it is exposed to the high CO_2 tensions generated by the fetus excreting CO_2. The CO_2 diffuses into the mother's red blood cells and dissociates as described. As the fetus offloads its CO_2 to its mother, who 'accepts' it, the fetus' curve moves left, while the maternal one moves right. This is called the 'double Bohr effect'.
> The fetal haemoglobin has a P_{50} of ~2.5 kP_a and so lies to the left of the mother's whose P_{50} is ~3.5 kP_a. This supports uptake of oxygen by the fetus.

How is the Haldane effect relevant to the placenta?

The Haldane effect describes the increased affinity of deoxygenated haemoglobin for CO_2 and vice versa. This is relevant across the placenta because as the fetus gives up CO_2 it increases its affinity for O_2, and as the mother gives up her O_2 her haemoglobin has an increased affinity for the CO_2. This is called the 'double Haldane effect'.

Describe the placental handling of the following anaesthetic drugs.

> **Thiopentone:** Crosses the placenta rapidly but the neonate does not suffer excessive sedation unless doses exceed 8 mg/kg.
> **Suxamethonium:** Does not cross the placenta in significant quantities unless the mother suffers from pseudocholinesterase deficiency, allowing significant concentrations to be present in her blood for a prolonged amount of time. The normally decreased levels of pseudocholinesterase found in pregnancy are not clinically significant.
> **Non-depolarising neuromuscular blockers:** These fully ionised, bulky, poorly lipid-soluble drugs do not cross the placenta.
> **Ephedrine:** Crosses easily.

39. FETAL CIRCULATION

The simplest way to tackle this subject is to draw this schematic diagram and use it in your subsequent discussion. This diagram looks busy at first, but don't be put off, it's very simple to draw after a few goes.

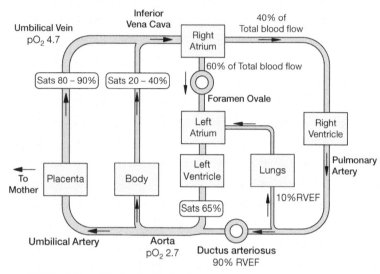

RVEF = right ventricular ejection fraction

Fig. 39.1 Schematic of fetal circulation

Can you describe the fetal circulation?

Talking it through, start at the placenta.

- Gas and waste exchange occurs at the placental bed. Oxygenated blood then flows from the placenta towards the fetus, via the umbilical vein.
- It enters the fetus and flows up the inferior vena cava to the right atrium.
- From here, ~60% of the blood flows through the foramen ovale, from right to left atrium. This blood travels from the left atrium to the left ventricle and from here is pumped out into the aorta to circulate to the brain, heart and body.
- The other 40% passes from the right atrium to the right ventricle. This ventricle contracts ejecting blood into the pulmonary artery. However, because of the high resistance afforded by the lungs, only 10% of this blood flows through the pulmonary bed; the other 90% follows the path of least resistance and flows through the ductus arteriosus to the descending aorta. Here, it joins the blood that originally flowed through the foramen ovale to left side of the heart.
- The blood continues its journey to and through the body, ultimately leaving the fetus to return to the placental bed, via the umbilical arteries, which arise from the common iliac arteries. (N.B. There are two umbilical arteries and one vein.)

How is preferential oxygenation to the major organs achieved?

- The pO_2 in the umbilical vein is only ~4.7 kP_a, representing saturations of 80–90%, and so the fetus is hypoxaemic when compared to the mother.
- Blood arriving in the right atrium from the inferior vena cava has saturations of ~60%, as it is composed of blood from the umbilical vein, mixed with deoxygenated blood returning from the body.
- The blood returning to the RA from the superior vena cava is even more deoxygenated, with sats of ~25%, because of the relatively high oxygen extraction of the brain. Clearly, it is sensible for this blood to be returned to the placental bed for re-oxygenation via as direct a route as possible, and certainly not to be re-introduced to the cerebral circulation. This is achieved by a structure called the Eustachian valve, a tissue flap found at the junction of the inferior vena cava and right atrium. It causes preferential 'streaming' of the more highly oxygenated inferior vena cava blood straight across the foramen ovale, to the left atrium to be expelled in to the aorta and therefore supply the brain. The less oxygenated blood of the superior vena cava 'falls' into the right ventricle to be distributed to the lungs and through the ductus arteriosus. This blood rejoins the aorta at a point distal to the origin of the carotids, therefore ensuring that the brain and heart are supplied with the most oxygen-rich blood.

Can you describe the changes that take place in the fetal circulation at birth?

Several things happen here, we think it's best to break it down in to stages when trying to explain it:

The gasp
As the baby is born it takes its first breath, often called a gasp. The generation of negative intrathoracic pressure alters Starling's forces across the pulmonary vessels and helps to reduce the amount of interstitial fluid in the lungs. A dramatic drop in pulmonary vascular resistance follows, allowing an increase in blood flow through the lungs. As a result, more blood returns to the left atrium from the lungs. This increases left-sided pressures in the heart, causing mechanical closure of the foramen ovale. So, yet more blood flows though the pulmonary bed as it now has no other path to go by, and this maintains the foramen ovale's closure.

Clamping the cord
As the cord is clamped, the ultra low-pressure placental circulation is removed from the baby. This causes a rise in systemic vascular resistance, and the removal of the blood from the placental circulation causes a reduction in venous return to the heart. This decreases right atrial filling pressures, therefore increasing further the pressure gradient between the left and right atria, helping further to keep the foramen ovale closed.

The ductus arteriosus
There is a net reduction in the amount of blood being shunted across the ductus arteriosus, as the pulmonary circulation is no longer a high-pressure system. The gradient between pulmonary vessels and the aorta is reversed, making the path through the lungs the one of least resistance.

In addition to this, the baby's blood now has a higher pO_2 than it did as a fetus. The movement of this more highly oxygenated blood across the ductus arteriosus stimulates its closure. The ductus arteriosus is closed physiologically at around 15 hours after birth, and anatomically by 15 days. Oxygen, bradykinins and prostaglandin antagonists (e.g. indomethacin) accelerate ductus arteriosus closure, while PGE1 (e.g. alprostdil) and conditions causing a raised pulmonary vascular resistance such as cold and acidosis help to keep it open. It is important therefore to keep neonates warm, oxygenated and hydrated (warm, wet and pink) to prevent their reverting to a fetal circulation, which can be disastrous as they obviously no longer have the ability to oxygenate themselves via a placenta.

40. AGEING

Approach this question using a systems-based technique. Remember that each elderly patient presenting for surgery is an amalgam of the presenting acute disease, the process of ageing and residual effects of any previous illness.

How does ageing alter physiology, and how does this impact on your anaesthetic practice?

Ageing is an irreversible process, which causes gradual reduction in the reserve of each system. The process affects everyone at different speeds, and often the decline is not obvious until almost total loss of reserve occurs. It is important to make a global assessment addressing physical, psychological and relevant social issues.

Cardiovascular system:
> Fewer pacemaker cells, making atrial fibrillation and other arrhythmias increasingly common with age. A pre-operative ECG is essential to look for any underlying pathology. The tendency towards bradycardia (sinus or otherwise) is exaggerated during general anaesthesia, so consider the use of anticholinergic agents such as glycopyrrolate.
> The compliance of the whole vascular system reduces. There is reduced compliance of the left ventricle, which hypertrophies in the face of increased afterload. Atherosclerosis is often present and contributes to the development of hypertension.
> Baroreceptor reflexes become less efficient with age and so compensation for a change in posture, for example is reduced, which can lead to hypotension. The tachycardic response is attenuated, and the elderly increase their cardiac outputs by increasing stroke volume, rather than heart rate. To try to minimise all these effects, aim to ensure adequate, but not overhydration prior to induction, and try to avoid rapid swings in blood pressure during induction and subsequent maintenance of anaesthesia. Hence, intravenous induction of anaesthesia using propofol should be slow, titrating the dose to effect, remembering that the arm–brain circulation time may be greatly increased.
> In addition to the effects of normal ageing, there may be other pathology such as ischaemic heart disease.

Respiratory system:
> ↓ pulmonary elasticity.
> ↓ chest wall and lung compliance.
> ↓ TLC, FEV1, FVC, IRV.
> ↑ RV.
> FRC is not altered but closing capacity gradually encroaches on it, and will exceed it, when supine, from around 65 years old.
> Upper airway tone and the cough reflex decrease, causing an increased risk of obstruction and airway soiling.
> The elderly are more prone to infections and pulmonary emboli, and the incidence of diseases such as COPD increases with age.
> In elective surgery it may be sensible to refer the patient to the respiratory physicians for pre-optimisation of any chest pathology.

Renal:

> The kidney's ability to both preserve and excrete water and electrolytes decreases.
> A reduction in muscle bulk is reflected in a decreased baseline creatinine.
> Careful attention to fluid balance, both peri- and post-operatively, is required.
> It is sensible to avoid NSAIDs in those with pre-existing renal failure, and to limit their use to 3 days in those with normal renal function.
> Be aware that a modest rise in creatinine level may reflect a significant decline in renal function.

Central nervous system:

> The acuity of the special senses (sight, hearing) decreases with age. This can lead to difficulties in communicating, and can increase confusion in the elderly.
> Confusion and dementia increase with age and can be exacerbated by anaesthesia.
> Cerebrovascular disease is common.
> Avoid intra-operative hypotension, which may result in cerebrovascular accident and attempt to avoid any centrally acting drugs that increase confusion where possible, e.g. atropine. It is sensible to try to recover confused patients in a quiet, calm, well-lit environment.

Musculoskeletal:

> Skin may be fragile. Extra care should be taken when moving the patient and attention to pressure areas to avoid the development of pressure sores.
> Arthritis is very common, and so care should be taken when positioning the anaesthetised patient so as not to cause pain in any affected joints. Pay special attention to neck mobility, especially in a patient with rheumatoid arthritis, looking specifically for the risk of atlanto-axial subluxation and a difficult airway.
> Balance, strength and postural reflexes worsen with age and so early mobilisation and physiotherapy is important to try to prevent significant loss of function in the post-operative period.

Pharmacology:

Pharmacokinetics can be altered due to:

> ↓ body fat and ↓ body water content.
> ↓ renal and liver blood flow.
> ↓ protein affects levels of free drug available.
> MAC ↓ with age.
> ↑ sensitivity to central depressants.
> Polypharmacy.
> Be cautious with dosing drugs with narrow therapeutic indices, e.g. gentamicin. It may be necessary to decrease the dose, or increase the time between consecutive doses.

41. ADRENAL GLAND

Questions on the adrenal gland should be relatively straightforward, but you will need a good understanding of the different endocrine feedback mechanisms that exist. Endocrine-based questions can also easily lead into clinical issues of under/overactive glands, so for this section we would recommend you familiarise yourself with hyperaldosteronism (primary and secondary), Addison's disease, Cushing's syndrome and phaeochromocytomas.

Describe the anatomical organisation of the adrenal gland.

The adrenal or suprarenal glands lie on top of the upper poles of the kidneys and play a key role in the synthesis of corticosteroids and catecholamines.

The adrenal glands are at the level of the twelfth thoracic vertebra. Anatomically, the adrenal gland is divided into two distinct areas: an outer cortex and inner medulla.

Adrenal cortex:
> Site of synthesis of corticosteroid hormones (glucocorticoids and mineralocorticoids) and androgens.
> Under neuroendocrine control via the hypothalamic–pituitary–adrenal axis.
> Part of the renin–angiotensin–aldosterone pathway.
> Divided into three functional zones from outside to inside: zona glomerulosa, zona fasciculata and zona reticularis (an easy way to remember this is 'GFR').

Adrenal medulla:
> Composed of chromaffin cells.
> Main site of synthesis of adrenaline and noradrenaline.
> Hormone secretion occurs in response to stimulation by pre-ganglionic (cholinergic) nerve fibres from the sympathetic nervous system (via splanchnic nerves).

What are the main hormones secreted from each of the three zones of the adrenal cortex?

> **Zona glomerulosa:** mineralocorticoids (aldosterone).
> **Zona fasciculata:** glucocorticoids (cortisol).
> **Zona reticularis:** androgens (dehydroepiandrosterone).

Describe the cortisol negative feedback pathway.

The hypothalamus secretes corticotrophin-releasing hormone (CRH), which stimulates release of adrenocorticotropic hormone (ACTH) from the anterior pituitary. ACTH stimulates cortisol secretion from the zona fasciculata of the adrenal cortex. Cortisol exerts negative feedback on both CRH and ACTH release.

Describe the control of aldosterone secretion.

> **Renin–angiotensin–aldosterone (RAA) system:** Reduced circulating volume is detected by the reduction in renal afferent arteriolar pressure causing renin secretion from the juxtaglomerular cells. Renin cleaves angiotensinogen to produce angiotensin I, which is then converted to angiotensin II in the pulmonary vasculature by angiotensin-converting enzyme (ACE). Angiotensin II promotes aldosterone secretion.
> **Fall in plasma sodium concentration:** Reduced serum sodium is detected by the macula densa in the distal convoluted tubule of the kidney and stimulates the secretion of aldosterone in order to increase sodium retention.
> **Rise in plasma ACTH:** Also exerts a direct effect in increasing aldosterone secretion from the zona glomerulosa.

What are major actions of cortisol?

Cortisol exerts its effects by binding to glucocorticoid receptors and promoting specific enzyme synthesis. The glucocorticoids works in many ways to provide resistance to 'stress', having effects on metabolism, immune function and vascular reactivity.

> **Metabolism:**
> • Increased protein catabolism
> • Increased hepatic gluconeogenesis and increased plasma glucose levels
> • Increased lipolysis

> **Vascular:**
> • Cortisol is essential in maintaining vascular reactivity to noradrenaline.

> **Immune:**
> • Suppresses the immune system, impairs wound healing and has anti-inflammatory effects.

What are the main actions of aldosterone?

Aldosterone increases the reabsorption of sodium from the distal convoluted tubules of the kidney, resulting in sodium retention and plasma expansion. It also increases urinary potassium excretion.

Describe how catecholamines are synthesised.

Catecholamines are synthesised in the chromaffin cells of the adrenal medulla:

L-TYROSINE

↓ Tyrosine hydroxylase

L-DOPA

↓ Dopa decarboxylase

DOPAMINE

↓ Dopamine hydroxylase

NORADRENALINE

↓ Phenylethanolamine *N*-methyltransferase

ADRENALINE

42. THYROID GLAND

Describe the structure of the thyroid gland.

The thyroid gland is a highly vascular structure made up of two lobes, joined together by the thyroid isthmus. The lobes are found on either side of the trachea, anterolaterally, below the larynx. The isthmus passes in front of the trachea overlying the second to fourth tracheal rings in the adult.

At a cellular level, the gland is made up of thousands of follicles. Each of these is made up of a single layer of cells surrounding a cavity. These epithelial cells make thyroid hormones and secrete them into the cavity, where they are stored bound to thyroglobulin, which is a globular colloidal substance.

What are the thyroid hormones and how are they made?

There are three different thyroid hormones:
> Thyroxine (T4)
> 3,5,3-Triiodothyronine (T3)
> 3,3,5-Triiodothyronine (reverse T3)

The majority of hormone synthesised is T4, but the active hormone is actually T3, which is five times more potent. T4 is converted to T3 peripherally to cause its biological effect. Reverse T3 is inactive.

T3/T4 are made as follows:

> The thyroid gland takes in iodine by active transport and concentrates it here.
> This iodine is oxidised to atomic iodine by peroxidase.
> The atomic iodine iodinates tyrosine residues found on the thyroglobulin molecule to form mono– or di-iodotyrosine.
> These iodinated tyrosine residues then couple up to form either T3 or T4.
> The T3 and T4 hormones are stored as an integral part of the thyroglobulin molecule.

This process is driven by thyroid-stimulating hormone (TSH) acting via cAMP. TSH also stimulates the release of the hormones by driving the endothelial cells to take in the colloidal thyroglobulin by pinocytosis. Once in the cell, proteolysis of the molecule causes release of T3 and T4. These diffuse into the ready blood supply and are transported out of the gland bound mainly to T4-binding globulin, but also to albumin and transthyretin.

What are the effects of the thyroid hormones?

T3, the major active hormone, exerts its effects by combining with a receptor in the cell nucleus and modulating protein synthesis at the level of the DNA. The actions of thyroid hormone can be divided into:

Metabolic
• Increased basal metabolic rate by increasing the rate of oxidative metabolism
• Increased sensitivity to catecholamines
• Increased breakdown of proteins, causing muscle wasting if unchecked
• Increased turnover of calcium from bone.

Growth
Needed for normal growth of tissues. Thyroid hormones exert a direct effect and also have a permissive effect on growth hormone.

Nervous system

Needed for development of the nervous system and normal myelination.

Others

Needed for normal gonadal function and for lactation.

How are thyroid hormone levels controlled?

The hypothalamus produces thyroid-releasing hormone, which stimulates the release of TSH from the anterior pituitary. This in turn causes the release of T4/T3 from the thyroid gland. The T4/T3 released exerts a negative feedback effect on the hypothalamus and pituitary thereby reducing further release of stimulating hormones.

Ultimately, T4/T3 are broken down in the liver and most tissues. T4 has a half-life of around 1 week, while T3's is much shorter at around 1 day.

What are the symptoms and signs of hyperthyroidism?

Table 42.1 Symptoms and signs of hyperthyroidism

System	Symptoms	Signs
CNS	Irritable, change in behaviour, anxiety, eye changes, goitre	Tremor, restless, irritable, frank psychosis in severe cases, goitre, hyper-reflexia. Eye signs: exophthalmos (Graves'), lid lag, ophthalmoplegia
CVS	Palpitations, racing heart	Tachycardia, atrial fibrillation, hypertension, high-output cardiac failure, warm and dilated peripheries
RS	Breathlessness	None specific
GI	Weight loss despite increased intake, vomiting, diarrhoea	Weight loss
GU	Loss of libido, gynaecomastia	Oligo/amenorrhoea, gynaecomastia
Musculoskeletal	Weakness, tremor, fatigue	Proximal muscle wasting, tremor, palmar erythema, pretibial myxoedema

What are the symptoms and signs of hypothyroidism?

Table 42.2 Symptoms and signs of hypothyroidism

System	Symptoms	Signs
CNS	Fatigue, slowness of thought	Flat affect, deafness, frank psychosis in severe cases, slow relaxing reflexes, ataxia
CVS	Ankle swelling	Bradycardia, ischaemic heart disease, peripheral oedema, low-output cardiac failure, pericardial effusion (rare), hypertension, vasoconstricted and cold peripheries
RS	None	None
GI	Weight gain	Weight gain, constipation
GU	Menorrhagia	Infertility
Musculoskeletal	Thinning of hair, loss of eyebrows, dry skin	Proximal myopathy, muscular hypertrophy, myotonia

43. EYE

Which cranial nerves supply the extraocular muscles?	Remember 'LR$_6$SO$_4$'. > Lateral rectus muscle is supplied by the sixth cranial nerve (abducens nerve). > Superior oblique muscle is supplied by the fourth cranial nerve (trochlear nerve). > All of the other extraocular muscles (medial rectus, superior rectus, inferior rectus and inferior oblique) are supplied by the third cranial nerve (oculomotor nerve).
What determines intraocular pressure (IOP)?	Intraocular pressure is normally less than 15mmHg. The effects of external pressure and the pressure exerted by intraocular contents (aqueous humour, choroidal blood volume and vitreous humour) determine the IOP.
What are the causes of raised IOP?	> **Increased extrinsic pressure**, e.g. retrobulbar haematoma, orbital compression in the prone position. > **Increased aqueous humour**, e.g. open-angle glaucoma (angle between iris and cornea remains patent but partially obstructed trabecular meshwork), closed-angle glaucoma (anterior bulging of the iris closing the drainage angle, trabecular meshwork remains patent). > **Sulphur hexafluoride injection**, e.g. during retinal surgery SF6 may be injected into the vitreous. Nitrous oxide interacts with SF6 by increasing the volume of the gas and therefore may increase IOP. > **Increased choroidal blood volume**, e.g. gravitational effects of head down position, hypoxia, hypercarbia, hypertension.
Describe the effects on IOP of the commonly used anaesthetic drugs.	> **Induction agents** – all agents except for ketamine lower IOP. > **Volatiles** – all lower IOP. > **N$_2$O** – has no effect on IOP unless used in combination with surgical use of SF6 during vitreo-retinal surgery. > **Neuromuscular blocking agents** – non-depolarising relaxants slightly lower IOP through reduction in extraocular muscle tension; suxamethonium causes a transient rise in IOP.
What is the oculocardiac reflex and how can it be prevented?	Oculocardiac reflex describes the bradycardia and or asystole observed as a result of traction on the extraocular muscles or extrinsic compression of the eye. The reflex pathway involves the trigeminal nerve and the vagus nerve. It is more pronounced in children. It may be obtunded by administration of anticholinergics such as atropine.

44. ENDOTHELIUM

What is the basic structure of endothelium?

Endothelium refers to the simple squamous epithelium that is found lining organs, blood vessels and body cavities. This single layer of cells lies on top of a basement membrane, and in small arteries, arterioles and glands it is also in proximity to smooth muscle. Endothelial structure varies according to its site and function. The major types include:

> **Continuous endothelium:** It consists of a continuous basement membrane with endothelial cells anchored together via tight junctions. It has a low permeability and is found in the blood–brain barrier and the lung.
> **Fenestrated endothelium:** It has pores (fenestrae) within the endothelium. It is very permeable and is found lining renal glomeruli.
> **Discontinuous endothelium:** It has large gaps between the endothelial cells and basement membrane. It is the most permeable of all types and is found in the liver and spleen.

What are the functions of endothelium?

Endothelium is a highly sophisticated and cellularly active tissue with essential roles in coagulation, inflammation and vasomotor tone. Its functions are varied and include the following:

> **Diffusion:** The endothelial lining at the alveolar–capillary interface plays an important role in the diffusion of gases (e.g. O_2 and CO_2) and lipid-soluble agents (e.g. anaesthetic drugs). The diffusion of such substances follows Fick's law.
> **Osmosis:** The endothelium lining the smaller blood vessels forms a semi-permeable membrane, which allows the formation of interstitial fluid, based on Starling's forces.
> **Filtration:** The pores present within the endothelium of the Bowman's capsule permit the passage of fluid and electrolytes via bulk flow and thereby enable blood to be filtered.
> **Barrier:** In the blood–brain barrier the tightly anchored endothelial cells form a relatively impermeable barrier that protects the central nervous system.
> **Vasomotor tone:** Endothelium releases several vasoactive substances that are crucial in regulating vascular smooth muscle tone. It produces nitric oxide (NO) from L-arginine in a reaction catalysed by nitric oxide synthetase. NO activates guanylate cyclase to produce cGMP, which causes vasodilatation. Endothelin-1 is another vasoactive substance produced by endothelial cells that causes vascular smooth muscle vasoconstriction.
> **Inflammation:** Vascular endothelium can synthesise several prostaglandins with prostacyclin (PGI_2) being the major derivative. PGI_2 promotes vasodilatation and inhibits platelet adhesion and therefore when vascular endothelium is damaged (e.g. atherosclerotic plaques) these vessels become prone to vasospasm and thrombosis.

> **Coagulation:** Endothelial damage exposes blood to tissue factor, which initiates the activation of the extrinsic clotting cascade.
> **Secretion:** Vascular endothelium, especially that lining the lungs, is rich in angiotensin-converting enzyme (ACE) that catalyses the conversion of angiotensin I to angiotensin II. This forms an important step in the renin–angiotensin–aldosterone system regulating blood pressure, sodium and water.

45. PORTAL CIRCULATIONS

What is the definition of a portal circulation?

A portal circulation is one in which blood from the capillary bed of one organ structure drains into the capillary bed of another organ structure through a larger vessel, usually a vein or venule (hence they are also known as portal venous systems).

Name some portal circulations?

Examples of such circulations include the hepatic portal (*see* Chapter 22, 'Liver physiology'), placental, hypothalamo-hypophyseal and renal circulations (*see* Chapter 27, 'Renal blood flow').

Describe the anatomical organisation of the pituitary gland.

The pituitary gland is a pea-shaped structure that lies within the sella turcica of the sphenoid bone. It is approximately 1–1.5 cm in diameter and is attached to the hypothalamus via the infundibulum. The pituitary gland is made up of two anatomically and functionally separate portions – the anterior pituitary (or adenohypophysis) and the posterior pituitary (or neurohypophysis).

The anterior pituitary:
> Synthesis and release of hormones is under the control of the hypothalamus.
> Hypothalamic hormones either stimulate or inhibit the release of hormones from the anterior pituitary.
> Hypothalamic hormones form an integral link between the nervous system and the endocrine systems.
> These hypothalamic hormones reach the anterior pituitary via portal blood vessels – the hypothalamo-hypophyseal portal circulation, which directly connect the two regions.
> This allows hormones synthesised by the hypothalamic neurones to be transported rapidly and directly to the anterior pituitary, avoiding dilution or destruction in the systemic circulation.
> These hormones diffuse into capillaries of the primary plexus (a capillary network located at the base of the hypothalamus) and are carried by hypophyseal portal veins (which run on the outside of the infundibulum) into the secondary capillary plexus of the anterior pituitary gland.

Posterior pituitary:
> It contains axons and axon terminals of over 10 000 neurosecretory cells whose cell bodies lie within the hypothalamus.
> These hypothalamic neurosecretory cells produce two hormones; oxytocin and antidiuretic hormone, ADH.
> Oxytocin and ADH are packed into vesicles and transported to the axon terminals in the posterior pituitary.
> Nerve impulses propagated along the axon trigger exocytosis of these vesicles and the released oxytocin and ADH then diffuse into the nearby capillaries.

What hormones are released by the hypothalamus?

Table 45.1   Actions of hypothalamic hormones

Hypothalamic hormones	Effects on anterior pituitary hormones
Growth hormone-releasing hormone (GHRH)	Stimulates release of growth hormone (GH)
Thyrotropin-releasing hormone (TRH)	Stimulates release of thyroid-stimulating hormone (TSH)
Gonadotropin-releasing hormone (GnRH)	Stimulates release of follicle-stimulating hormone (FSH) and luteinising hormone (LH)
Corticotropin-releasing hormone (CRH)	Stimulates release of adenocorticotropic hormone (ACTH) and melanocyte-stimulating hormone (MSH)
Prolactin-releasing hormone (PRH)	Stimulates release of prolactin

What are the effects of the anterior pituitary hormones?

Table 45.2   The effects of anterior pituitary hormones

Anterior pituitary hormone	Effect
GH	Stimulates liver to synthesise and release insulin-like growth factors (IGFs). These stimulate protein anabolism, lipolysis, tissue repair, cell growth and elevate plasma glucose levels
TSH	Stimulates thyroid gland to release thyroxine (T4) and triiodothyronine (T3).
FSH	In females stimulates production of oocytes and secretion of ovarian oestrogen. In males stimulates sperm production.
LH	In females, stimulates ovulation, corpus luteum formation, secretion of ovarian oestrogen and secretion of corpus luteum progesterone. In males stimulates secretion of testicular testosterone.
ACTH	Stimulates release of glucocorticoids (mainly cortisol) from the adrenal cortex.
MSH	Stimulates darkening of skin.
Prolactin	Stimulates milk production.

What is the effect of ADH release on the body?

This is covered in Chapter 30, 'Fluid compartments'.

Describe the renal portal circulation.

The kidney is interesting because it contains two portal circulations. An afferent arteriole enters the Bowman's capsule and divides into multiple capillaries to form the glomerulus (this is the primary capillary bed). The efferent venule leaving the glomerulus enters two distinct secondary capillary beds: a capillary bed surrounding the cortical tubular system and a capillary bed surrounding the loop of Henle (the vasa recta). The function of these portal circulations is to maximise the reabsorption of water and electrolytes filtered at the glomerulus.

46. IMMUNE MECHANISMS

What types of immunity are there?

The immune system comprises a system of cellular and non-cellular biological mechanisms that defend an organism against disease.

Immunity can be classified as **non-specific (or innate)** and **specific (or acquired/adaptive)**.

Both types depend on the immune system's ability to distinguish between self-and non-self-molecules. Both types consist of humoral and cell-mediated components.

The non-specific immune system does not recognise the substance that is being attacked, but responds against pathogens in a generic way, and does not confer long-lasting immunity against pathogens. It is present from birth.

Specific immunity is antigen specific and requires the recognition of non-self-antigens during a process called antigen presentation. It confers immunological memory by the action of memory cells.

Non-specific/innate immunity
> **Surface barriers:**
  - Mechanical: skin, coughing and sneezing expels organisms; tears and urine flush away pathogens; mucus traps organisms
  - Chemical: antibacterial enzymes in tears, saliva and breastmilk; hostile acidic environment of stomach
  - Biological: lower GIT bacterial flora that prevents overgrowth of pathogenic bacteria.

> **Inflammatory response:**
  - One of the first responses to infection or injury, mediated by eicosanoids and cytokines.
  - Eicosanoids produce prostaglandins, which cause fever and blood vessel dilation, and leukotrienes, which attract white blood cells (WBC) to the site of infection.
  - Cytokines include interleukins (communication between WBC), chemokines (chemotaxis) and interferons (antiviral activity).
  - The symptoms of inflammation are redness, swelling, heat and pain, caused by increased blood flow to the site of injury/infection.

> **Activation of the alternative complement pathway:**
  - Complement is a biochemical enzyme system comprising more than 20 glycoproteins that, when activated, result in a rapid catalytic cascade and eventual target cell lysis.
  - The complement cascade results in opsonisation (coating) of target cells and disruption of their cell membrane phospholipids, attraction of immune cells, and increased vascular permeability.
  - The classical complement pathway is a specific immune response and involves the binding of complement to antibodies on the surface of pathogens.
  - The alternative complement pathway is a non-specific immune response and involves the binding of complement to carbohydrates on the surface of microbes, but also to bacterial toxins and certain drugs.

> **Phagocytosis:**
> - The leucocytes involved in innate immunity include neutrophils (50–70%), macrophages, monocytes (2–6%), eosinophils (1–6%), basophils (1%), mast cells and natural killer (NK) lymphocytes.
> - Phagocytosis is the process of ingestion of a microorganism, another cell or cell fragments by a phagocyte to form an intracellular phagosome. This fuses with a lysosome, which in turn releases lysozymes, which digest the particle.
> - Neutrophils are usually the first cells to arrive at the site of infection, and aside form phagocytosis, they also release inflammatory mediators.
> - Macrophages are abundant within tissues and act as scavengers of worn-out cells and destroyers of foreign material by both phagocytosis and extracellular release of toxic chemicals. They also release cytokines (interleukins, interferon, tumour necrosis factor) and complement protein, and activate the adaptive immune system by acting as antigen-presenting cells (APC).
> - Monocytes are the circulatory equivalent of macrophages.
> - Basophils are the circulatory equivalent of mast cells, both of which release histamines in response to allergens.
> - Eosinophils destroy parasites by extracellular release of enzymatic granules, and they may mediate hypersensitivity reactions.
> - NK cells are lymphocytes that destroy tumour cells and cells infected by viruses.

Specific Immunity

Specific immunity is so called because it is antigen specific. This allows for a stronger immune response that confers immunological memory for specific pathogens.

The major components include T and B lymphocytes, plasma cells, antibodies, the classic complement pathway, and immunological memory.

B lymphocytes are involved in humoral immunity and T lymphocytes in cell-mediated immunity. Both T and B lymphocytes have receptors that recognise specific antigenic targets.

> **T lymphocytes**
> - There are two major subtypes: helper T and killer T cells.
> - Another subtype, suppressor T cells, is involved in modulation of the immune response.
> - T cells recognise pathogens only after antigens (small, processed fragments of pathogens) bind to specific receptors (known as MHC, or major histocompatibility complex) on the surface of APC (e.g. macrophages).
> - T cell receptors bind to this antigen–MHC complex with the help of a co-receptor (CD4 on helper T cells and CD8 on killer T cells).
> - Killer T cells bind to antigen–MHC class 1, and helper T cells to antigen–MHC class 2.
> - After binding to the antigen complex, T cells become activated and begin to proliferate, some of which branch into memory cells.
> - Activated killer T cells release cytotoxins, which results in apoptosis of the host cell.
> - Activated helper T cells release cytokines that activate killer T cells, B lymphocytes and macrophages.

> **B lymphocytes and antibodies**
> - Antibodies on the surface of B cells bind to specific antigens. The Ag–Ab complex is taken up by the B cell and lysed, forming antigenic peptides that are then presented, bound to MHC 2 on the B cell surface.
> - This complex is recognised by helper T cells that release lymphokines, which in turn activate the B cell.

- Activated B cells proliferate forming other B cells, plasma cells and memory cells.
- Plasma cells are mostly found in lymph nodes, spleen and bone marrow. They produce and release millions of copies of antibodies into the circulation.
- Antibodies bind to antigen expressed on pathogens, marking them for destruction by either phagocytosis or the classic complement pathway.
- They can also bind directly to bacterial toxins and modulate receptors on host cells so that viruses and bacteria cannot penetrate them.
- Antibodies are composed of two heavy chains and two light chains, with a variable region at one end, allowing them to recognise their specific antigens.
- There are five main subtypes of antibody: IgG (most abundant), IgM (crucial in initial immune response), IgE (response to parasites and allergies), IgA (present in body fluids) and IgD (on cell surface of B lymphocytes).

What type of hypersensitivity reactions do you know?

Hypersensitivity reactions are abnormal immune responses, including allergies and autoimmunity, that damage the body's own tissues. Reactions occur on second or repeated exposure to the antigen involved.

They can be classified into four groups based on mechanism:

> **Type 1 (immediate, or anaphylactic)**
  This is the classic atopic/allergic response and occurs when IgE antibodies on the surface of mast cells and basophils bind to drug antigen. This causes the cells to degranulate, releasing histamines, serotonin, leukotrienes, platelet-activating factor and heparin into the circulation. These mediators cause vasodilatation, increased capillary permeability, increased secretion of mucus and smooth muscle spasm. The reaction occurs less than 1 hour from exposure. The most common peri-operative culprits include neuromuscular blockers, latex, antibiotics, dyes and NSAIDs.

> **Type 2 (antibody-dependent cytotoxic hypersensitivity)**
  Circulating IgE and IgM bind to antigen and activate macrophages, NK cells and the classic complement pathway, resulting in target cell lysis. Examples include blood transfusion reactions, erythroblastosis fetalis, autoimmune haemolytic anaemia, hyper-acute graft rejection of a transplanted organ, heparin-induced thrombocytopenia type 2, Graves' disease and myasthenia gravis.

> **Type 3 (immune-complex mediated)**
  Circulating antigen–antibody complexes deposit in vessels and tissues and activate the classic complement pathway. They may also activate the release of inflammatory mediators. Type 3 reactions typically occur 4–10 days after exposure to antigen and can become chronic. Many autoimmune diseases fall in this category: serum sickness, systemic lupus erythematosus, rheumatoid arthritis, and the glomerulonephritides (including post-streptococcal).

> **Type 4 (delayed)**
  This is a cell-mediated immune response, not involving antibodies or complement. T cells previously sensitised to an antigen become activated on re-exposure and can damage tissue either by direct toxic effects or by releasing cytokines that attract phagocytes to the area. Reactions typically take 24–48 hours to occur. Disorders of this type include contact dermatitis (including a reaction to the chemicals used in the production process of latex gloves), chronic transplant rejection, and the immune response to TB (including the tuberculin test in previously exposed individuals).

47. PAIN PATHWAYS

Define and classify pain.

Pain is 'an unpleasant sensory and emotional experience associated with actual or potential tissue damage'. (IASP: International Association for the Study of Pain)

Pain can be classified according to its chronicity:

> **Acute**
> • Recent onset, limited duration
> • Identifiable cause related to injury/disease

> **Chronic**
> • Persists beyond time of healing or injury
> • No clearly definable cause

It may also be classified according to its nature:

> **Nociceptive:** noxious stimulation of nociceptors. This may further be subdivided into:

  • Superficial somatic pain (skin) – well-localised, sharp pain
  • Deep somatic pain (ligaments, tendons, muscles) – dull aching poorly localised pain
  • Visceral pain (organs, viscera) – cramping pain, varying localisation, associated with referred pain and autonomic stimulation.

> **Neuropathic:** due to dysfunction of the nervous system.

Give a detailed description of the pain pathways that become activated if you prick your finger with a pin.

> Nociceptors respond to noxious stimuli, which may be thermal, mechanical or chemical.
> Tissue damage releases mediators, which initiate and sensitise receptor stimulation.
> An action potential is generated and propagated along the primary afferent nerve fibres (C & Aδ) to the dorsal horn of the spinal cord.
> Synaptic transmission with secondary interneurones occurs in Rexed's laminae.
> Secondary interneurones decussate and travel in the anterolateral spinothalamic tracts through the brainstem to the thalamus.
> From here, tertiary afferents project to the somatosensory cortex.
> Some spinal ascending fibres transmit impulses to the reticular-activating system, and to higher centres involved with affect, emotion and memory.
> Descending fibres from cortex, thalamus and brainstem exert an inhibitory influence on pain transmission in the dorsal horn
> An immediate polysynaptic withdrawal reflex occurs at the level of the spinal cord as some interneurones connect to motor neurones at many levels. This is a protective reflex.

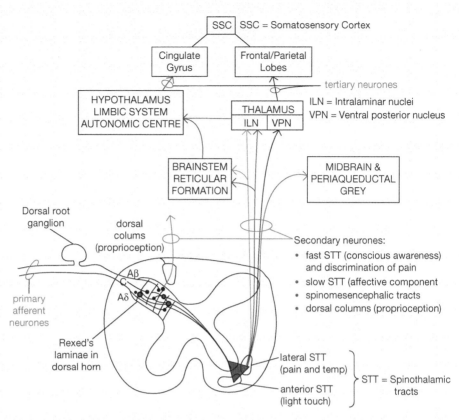

Fig. 47.1 Schematic representation of pain pathways

What are nociceptors and how are they classified?

Pain receptors are unmyelinated nerve endings that are abundant in skin and musculoskeletal tissue, and that respond to thermal, mechanical and chemical stimuli.

They are classified according to their sensitivity to the type of stimulus:

> **Unimodal** (thermo-mechanoreceptors) respond to pinprick and sudden heat.
> **Polymodal** respond to pressure, heat, cold, chemicals and tissue damage.

How do noxious stimuli activate pain transmission?

> Chemical stimuli may be exogenous (e.g. capsaicin) or endogenous.
> Tissue injury causes damage to cell membranes and release of endogenous chemicals, which stimulate nociceptors (bradykinin, histamine, serotonin, acetylcholine, H^+ and K^+ ions).
> Some chemical mediators lower the threshold for receptor stimulation, i.e. they sensitise nociceptors (prostaglandins, leukotrienes, substance P, neurokinin A and calcitonin gene-related peptide).
> Stimulation results in an influx of sodium and calcium ions, which causes depolarisation of the cell membrane and initiation of an action potential (AP).
> The AP is propagated along the nerve fibre (via sodium and calcium channels) to the dorsal root ganglion and the dorsal horn. The more heavily myelinated the nerve fibre is, the faster the impulse transmits.
> At the presynaptic terminal, the influx of calcium causes release of neurotransmitter into the synaptic cleft.

Which types of nerve fibres are involved?

> Three main types of fibres relay sensory inputs from the periphery (Table 47.1).
> The cell bodies of all three fibres lie in the dorsal root ganglia.
> The fibres terminate in the dorsal horn of the spinal cord, where they synapse with secondary afferent neurones in Rexed's laminae.

Table 47.1 Characteristics of different nerve fibres

Afferent fibres	Aβ	Aδ	C
Stimulus	Non-noxious (pressure/touch)	Non-noxious and noxious (pain and temperature)	Polymodal noxious (mechanical, heat, chemical)
Diameter (μm)	Large, 6–20	Small, 2–5	Small, 0.4–1.2
Myelin	Thick	Thin	No
Conduction velocity (ms⁻¹)	80–120	12–30	0.5–2
Type of pain	Touch, pressure (no pain)	Fast, sharp, well-localised	Diffuse, dull
Dorsal horn termination (Rexed's laminae)	III	I (superficial) & V (deep)	II & III (substantia gelatinosa)

What happens at the level of the dorsal horn?

> The dorsal horn is the area of synaptic transmission between primary and secondary afferent neurones in Rexed's laminae.
> Laminae II and III are called the substantia gelatinosa where extensive modulation of pain occurs. It is the site of the 'gate control' theory of pain.

Describe the classes of second-order neurones.

Table 47.2 Classes of second-order neurones

Class	Nociceptive-specific (NS)	Wide dynamic range (WDR)	Low-threshold neurones
Location	Superficial laminae	Deeper laminae	Laminae III and IV
Response to type of stimulus	Specific noxious	Non-specific	Innocuous
Synapse with primary fibre	C & Aδ	Aδ	Some Aβ

Which neurotransmitters and receptors are involved?

> The main excitatory neurotransmitters released by the primary afferent terminals include glutamate, aspartate and substance P ('glutam**ate** and aspart**ate** excit**ate**!'). These trigger various receptors on interneurones and secondary afferent neurones, such as:
> • N-Methyl-d-aspartate (NMDA)
> • α-Amino-3-hydroxy-5-methylisoxazole-4-propionic acid (AMPA)
> • Neurokinin-1 (NK1)
> • Adenosine (A1/A2)
> Inhibitory neurotransmitters released locally include:
> • Enkephalins (MOP opioid receptors)
> • Gamma-aminobutyric acid (GABA receptors).

Describe the path of the ascending spinal tracts to higher centres.

There are multiple ascending tracts. The most important ones are:

> **Spinothalamic tracts** (STT)
> • Most secondary fibres decussate and ascend as the anterolateral STT.
>   o Anterior STT: light touch.
>   o Lateral STT: pain and temperature.
> • Fast (discriminatory) and slow (affective) fibres travel together to the brainstem where they separate to end in different nuclei.
> • Fast fibres pass through the brainstem with no intermediary synapses before terminating in the ventral posterior nucleus of the thalamus. From here, tertiary neurones project to the somatosensory cortex (parietal and frontal lobes). They are responsible for conscious perception and memory of pain as well as its discrimination (location, intensity, quality).

- Slow (affective) fibres synapse in the brainstem's reticular formation and in intralaminar nuclei of the thalamus before projecting to the hypothalamus, limbic system and autonomic centres.
- Tertiary fibres project to the cingulate gyrus in the cortex. They are associated with the affective-arousal component of pain.

> **Spinoreticular tracts**
- Slow fibres may also ascend in the spinoreticular tract, terminating in the reticular formation and thalamus.

> **Spinomesencephalic tracts**
- These terminate in the midbrain and periaqueductal grey (PAG).

> **Dorsal columns**
- Pressure, vibration and proprioception carried by Aβ fibres from the periphery ascend in the dorsal columns ipsilaterally.
- They do not transmit pain sensation to higher centres.

Describe the descending inhibitory pathways.

> **Periaqueductal grey** (PAG) in the midbrain.
- This is the main descending pathway.
- It receives projections from the thalamus, hypothalamus, amygdala and cortex, and delivers projections to the nucleus raphe magnus (NRM) in the medulla, whose fibres synapse in the substantia gelatinosa of the dorsal horn.
- Its transmitters include endorphins and enkephalins (MOP opioid receptors) and serotonin (5HT1 and 5HT3 receptors).

> **Locus caeruleus** (LC).
- An important brainstem nucleus projecting descending inhibitory pathways to the dorsal horn via noradrenaline (α-adrenergic receptors).

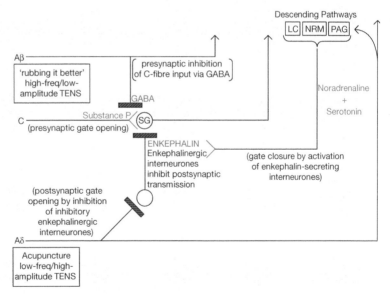

Fig. 47.2 'Gate Control' theory of pain

What do you understand by the 'gate control' theory of pain modulation?
(Melzack and Wall 1965)

> This is one aspect of pain modulation, reducing the response to nociceptive stimuli.
> It postulates that pain transmission from primary to secondary afferents is 'gated' by interneurones in the substantia gelatinosa.
> Inhibition can be presynaptic on primary afferents or postsynaptic on secondary afferent neurones.
>   • **Opening:** The 'gate' is opened presynaptically by C fibres via substance P ('pushes' the gate open) and postsynaptically by Aδ fibres, which inhibit the action of enkephalinergic interneurones (which are inhibitory) at the level of the substantia gelatinosa, thus allowing transmission of pain signals.
>   • **Closure:** It is closed by descending inhibitory fibres, peripheral Aβ fibres and indirectly by the action of Aδ fibres on descending pathways, which result in reduced transmission of pain signals.
>
> Aβ fibres inhibit C fibre input presynaptically via stimulation of GABA receptors (which are inhibitory). Aβ fibres are stimulated by touch/ pressure and explain how 'rubbing it better' and how high-frequency, low-amplitude TENS may attenuate pain.
> Descending serotonergic (PAG, NRM) and noradrenergic (LC) fibres activate enkephalin-secreting interneurones, which inhibit postsynaptic transmission. This explains how antidepressants (which block the reuptake of serotonin and noradrenaline) and opioids exert their effect.
> Aδ fibres ascend and stimulate the PAG to exert its inhibitory action as above. This explains how acupuncture and how low-frequency TENS may attenuate pain.

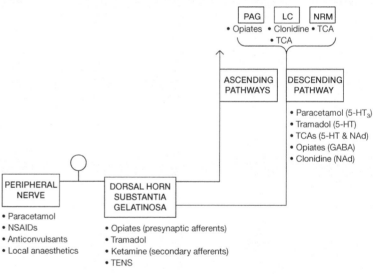

Fig. 47.3 Sites of action of analgesics

Where are the sites of action of commonly used analgesic methods?

Table 47.3 Sites of action of analgesics

Analgesic	Site of action	Receptor	Neurotransmitter
Paracetamol	Central	+ 5HT3 + Cannabinoid	+ Serotonin + Endogenous cannabinoids
	Peripheral	– COX	– Prostaglandins
NSAID	Nociceptor	– COX	– Prostaglandins
Opiate	DH (presynaptic afferents)	+ MOP opioid	Reduced glutamate release from Aδ & C fibres (reduced nociceptive transmission)
	Descending pathways: PAG (postsynaptic secondary afferents)	– GABA receptor	– GABA (increased anti-nociceptive transmission, i.e. GABAergic inhibition activates serotonergic and noradrenergic descending pathways)
Tramadol/ Pethidine	DH	+ MOP opioid	Reduced glutamate release from Aδ & C fibres
Tramadol/ Pethidine	Descending pathways	+ 5HT1 & 5HT3	Inhibition of reuptake of serotonin and noradrenaline
Tramadol	Descending pathways	+ α-Adrenergic + 5HT1 & 5HT3	+ Presynaptic serotonin release
Antidepressants (TCAs)	Descending pathways: • NRM • LC	+ 5HT1 & 5HT3 + α-Adrenergic	+ Serotonin + Noradrenaline (by inhibition of reuptake)
Anticonvulsants (phenytoin, carbamazepine, sodium valproate)	Peripheral nerves	Stabilise sodium channels	
Gabapentin (antinociceptive)	DH	Bind (block) to voltage-gated calcium channels	Inhibit release of excitatory glutamate, aspartate, substance P
	Descending pathways	Promotes noradrenaline-mediated inhibition	+ Noradrenaline
Local anaesthetics	Peripheral nerve fibre	Block sodium channels	
Ketamine	Dorsal horn secondary afferent	– NMDA	– Glutamate
Clonidine	LC	+ α2-Adrenergic agonist	+ Noradrenaline
TENS	Aβ fibres 'closing the gate' in dorsal horn by presynaptic inhibition	+ GABA	+ GABA

48. MUSCLE ELECTROPHYSIOLOGY

What is the resting membrane potential of a skeletal muscle cell?

Resting membrane potential for skeletal muscle is –90 mV, nervous tissue is –70 mV and cardiac muscle is –90 mV.

Describe the anatomical structure of a skeletal muscle.

A skeletal muscle is covered by a connective tissue called the epimysium. Within the muscle lie thousands of muscle fibres, which are arranged in bundles or fascicles, surrounded by perimysium. These muscle fibres are cylindrical, multi-nucleated cells, 10–100 μm in diameter and run along the entire length of the muscle. They are surrounded by endomysium.

Microscopically, muscle fibres have a striated appearance due to the presence of numerous myofibrils. The myofibrils are formed by thick (myosin) and thin (actin) contractile filaments in association with the regulatory proteins tropomyosin and troponin. These contractile filaments are arranged within sarcomeres, which form the basic contractile unit of a skeletal muscle.

What are the major components of the neuromuscular junction?

Neuromuscular transmission occurs across the neuromuscular junction, which is composed of the α-motor neurone, synaptic cleft and motor end plate of the muscle fibre.

The end terminals of the motor neurone are unmyelinated, with specialised sites for the storage and release of acetylcholine (ACh). The motor end plate of the muscle fibre is deeply folded, with high concentrations of nicotinic acetylcholine receptors (nAChR) located at the crests of these folds. Separating these two components is the synaptic cleft, a 20 μm gap containing acetylcholinesterase.

How is acetylcholine synthesised and stored within the nerve terminal?

ACh is synthesised within the axoplasm from choline (obtained from the diet and liver synthesis) and acetyl coenzyme A (a metabolic by-product) in a reaction catalysed by choline-O-acetyltransferase. Once formed, approximately 80% is stored in vesicles available for release. Some of these vesicles (about 1%) lie at special release sites known as 'active zones' and are available for immediate release, while the others form the 'reserve pool', and are ready for transportation to the release site when needed. A remaining 20% forms a 'stationary store' dissolved in the cytoplasm.

How does neuromuscular transmission occur?

When a motor nerve is depolarised, voltage-gated Ca^{2+} channels open in the presynaptic membrane, allowing Ca^{2+} to enter the nerve terminal. This Ca^{2+} enables the vesicles to fuse and release their contents, it is believed, by exocytosis.

Approximately 100–200 vesicles simultaneously release their ACh, producing an end-plate potential. When ACh binds to nAChR (pentameric, ligand-gated ion-channels consisting of 2α, 1β, 1ε and 1δ subunits) the receptor undergoes a conformational change and the central ion channel opens sufficiently to allow the passage of cations, predominantly Na^+ and K^+. This causes a localised depolarisation of the muscle fibre membrane, which leads to excitation–contraction coupling. The action of ACh is rapidly terminated by the presence of acetylcholinesterase within the synaptic cleft.

When do extra-junctional nAChR appear?

Extra-junctional nAChR rapidly sprout after denervation and burns injuries. These receptors are structurally different as the normal ε subunit is replaced by the fetal γ subunit. They are extremely sensitive to depolarising neuromuscular blocking agents and the use of these agents can result in profound hyperkalaemia. This is why suxamethonium is typically contraindicated in such patients from 24 hours to 2 years after injury. In contrast, extra-junctional receptors are relatively resistant to non-depolarising neuromuscular blocking agents and therefore these drugs must be administered at higher doses.

Describe the positive feedback mechanism designed to increase ACh release.

There are pre-junctional nAChR located on the nerve terminals, which form a positive feedback mechanism designed to increase the release of ACh during periods of high activity (e.g. tetanic stimulation). These receptors are blocked by non-depolarising neuromuscular blocking drugs and this explains why fade on train-of-four stimulation is observed with these agents.

What is a motor unit?

A motor unit refers to a single motor neurone and all the muscle fibres it innervates. In muscles involved in fine, precise movement (e.g. eyes and fingers) the motor units are small and one motor neurone innervates only a few muscle fibres. This is in sharp contrast to muscles involved in gross, powerful movement where the motor unit consists of a single neurone innervating hundreds of fibres (e.g. quadriceps muscle).

What is excitation–contraction coupling?

This refers to the process by which the electrical activity of muscle depolarisation results in mechanical changes leading to contraction.

As the action potential travels down the T-tubules, which lie very close to the sarcoplasmic reticulum, it triggers calcium release channels (i.e. the ryanodine receptors) on the sarcoplasmic reticulum to open, resulting in an influx of intracellular Ca^{2+}. This Ca^{2+} binds onto troponin, bringing about a conformational change in the troponin–tropomyosin complex, which results in the exposure of the myosin binding sites on the actin filaments. The myosin heads bind to actin and perform a ratchet-type movement towards the centre of the sarcomeres, dubbed 'the power stroke'. ATP then binds onto the myosin head, allowing it to detach from the actin. The hydrolysis of this ATP enables the myosin head to re-orientate itself ready for the next power stroke. The muscle relaxes when intracellular Ca^{2+} levels decrease.

Rigor mortis occurs due to the lack of ATP, which prevents the detachment of the myosin heads from actin and hence the filaments are held in sustained contraction.

In malignant hyperpyrexia there is a defect in the ryanodine receptor, which leads to the uncontrolled release of Ca^{2+} from within the sarcoplasmic reticulum and hence the sustained muscle contraction and rigidity seen in this condition.

49. REFLEXES

What are reflexes?

Reflexes are neuronal pathways that produce rapid, automatic and predictable responses to a stimulus. The basic components of the reflex arc include a receptor, afferent sensory neurone, synapse, efferent motor neurone and effector organ.

When we talk about reflexes we typically think of somatic reflexes, e.g. knee jerk stretch reflex, which are important in the functioning of the skeletal muscle system. However, equally important are the visceral reflexes, e.g. pupillary light reflex, which form the basis of the functioning of the autonomic nervous system.

What is the Bell–Magendie law?

This law states that the anterior spinal nerve roots contain only motor fibres and the posterior nerve roots contain only sensory fibres.

Describe the physiology of the stretch reflex.

The stretch reflex (e.g. knee jerk stretch reflex) is a monosynaptic reflex that results in the contraction of a muscle in response to its being stretched.

Muscle spindle receptors within the muscle are stimulated when the muscle fibres are stretched, resulting in the generation of an electrical potential. Provided this is of sufficient magnitude, an action potential is generated and propagates down afferent sensory neurones (Ia and II) to enter the grey matter of the spinal cord. They synapse within the ventral horn with efferent motor neurones (Aα), which project back to the extrafusal muscle fibres of the stretched muscle and cause it to contract. The sensory neurones also synapse with inhibitory inter-neurones, which innervate the antagonistic muscle group. Hence when the stretched muscle contracts during the reflex, its antagonistic muscles relax. This is known as reciprocal innervation. Stretch reflexes help maintain muscle tone, aid posture and prevent injury by opposing overstretching of muscles.

What is the inverse stretch reflex?

This refers to the relaxation of a muscle in response to a strong stretch. The harder a muscle is stretched, the more forcefully it will contract. However, there comes a point when muscle tension becomes so great that the Golgi tendon organs detect this and inhibit the activity of the efferent Aα motor neurones via an inhibitory feedback mechanism. This system is designed to prevent muscle damage.

Describe the physiology of the withdrawal (flexor) reflex.

This is an important reflex governing the response to a painful stimulus and is an example of a polysynaptic reflex. Nociceptors are stimulated and impulses are propagated along sensory Aδ and C fibres into the grey matter of the spinal cord. Here they synapse with inter-neurones that extend to several spinal cord segments. These inter-neurones activate various Aα motor neurones, which culminate in the contraction of the flexor muscles of the affected limb. However, in order to maintain balance during a sudden flexor withdrawal of a lower limb, the pain stimulus also activates a cross-extensor reflex, which results in the automatic extension of the contralateral limb.

How are nerve fibres classified?

Classification of nerve fibres has become confusing with the use of both alphabetical and numerical classification systems. Originally, mammalian nerves were classified alphabetically into A, B or C fibre types. The A fibre type was then further subdivided into α, β, γ and δ groups. However, as science evolved it became apparent that the alphabetical classification system was inadequate because not all nerve fibre types within the originally assigned group were the same. Therefore, a numerical system was introduced to classify sensory neurones.

Table 49.1 Classification of nerve fibres

Fibre type	Axon diameter (μm)	Velocity (m/s)	Function
Aα	10–20	60–120	Motor
Aβ	5–10	40–70	Touch Pressure
Aγ	3–6	15–30	Motor to muscle spindles
Aδ	2–5	10–30	Pain Temperature
B	1–3	3–15	Autonomic (pre-ganglionic)
C	0.5–1	0.5–2	Pain Temperature
Ia (Aα type)	12–20	72–120	Sensory from muscle spindle (annulospiral)
Ib (Aα type)	12–20	72–120	Sensory from Golgi tendon
II (Aβ type)	4–12	24–72	Sensory from muscle spindle (flower-spray)
III (Aδ type)	1–4	6–24	Pain Cold
IV (C type)	0.5–1	0.5–2	Pain Temperature

Part 02

PHYSICS

50. DEFINITIONS

Many of the physics SOEs will start with a definition, which will then lead on to more detailed questioning on the surrounding concepts. This list is by no means exhaustive and should you encounter other definitions it is worthwhile making note of them.

Absolute humidity:
> The mass of water vapour present in a particular sample of air at a given temperature.
> Measured as kg m^{-3}.

Absolute zero:
> The lowest possible temperature where nothing could be colder and all thermal motion stops.
> Precisely 0 K or −273.15 °C.

Ampere (A): SI unit of electric current (SI base unit)
> The current that produces a force of 2×10^{-7} newtons per metre between two parallel wires, of infinite length, 1 m apart in a vacuum.
> The ampere is a measure of the amount of electrical charge passing a given point per unit time.
> An equivalent charge to 6.24×10^{18} electrons (1 coulomb) per second = 1 ampere.

Boiling point:
> The temperature at which the vapour pressure of a liquid equals the surrounding ambient pressure and the liquid changes into a vapour.

Calorie:
> The amount of energy required to increase the temperature of 1 g of water by 1 °C.
> 1 calorie = 4.16 J.
> Kcalorie = Abbreviation for kilocalorie which = 1 large calorie (C) or 1000 small calories (c) or 4.16 kJ.

Candela (cd): The SI unit of luminous intensity (SI base unit).
> 1 cd is the luminous intensity, in a given direction, of a source that emits monochromatic radiation of frequency 540×10^{12} hertz and that has a radiant intensity in that direction of 1/683 watt per steradian.
> A normal candle emits light with a luminous intensity of roughly 1 candela.

Coulomb (C): The unit of charge.
> 1 C is the amount of charge passing a given point per second, when 1 A of current is flowing (*see* definition of Ampere above).
> 1 C = 1A × 1s.
> 1 C is the magnitude of charge possessed by 6.24×10^{18} electrons.

Critical temperature:
> The temperature above which a gas cannot be liquefied by pressure alone.

Freezing point:
> The temperature at which the liquid and solid phases of a substance of specified composition are in equilibrium at a given pressure.
> A liquid turns into a solid when its temperature is lowered below its freezing point.

Force:
> That which changes a body's state of rest or motion.
> Derived SI unit = the newton (N).
> 1N is the force required to accelerate a 1kg mass at a rate of 1m per second squared ($1N = 1$ kg·m·s^{-2}).
> Force has both magnitude and direction, making it a vector.
> Force = mass × acceleration ($F = ma$).

Gas:
> One of the four fundamental states of matter found between the liquid and plasma phase (four states = solid, liquid, gas and plasma).
> A substance which is above its critical temperature.
> It is distinguished from liquids and solids by the vast separation between individual gas particles.
> A gas will expand to fill any space available.

Heat capacity:
> The amount of heat required to raise the temperature of an object by 1 °C (specific heat capacity × mass of body).
> SI unit of heat capacity = joule per kelvin.

Hertz (Hz): Derived SI unit of frequency
> 1 Hz is 1 cycle per second.

Joule (J): Derived SI unit of energy
> 1 J is the work done (or energy expended) to an object when applying of a force of 1 newton through a distance of 1 m.
> $1J = 1N \times 1m$ or 1 newton metre.

Kelvin (K): SI unit of temperature (SI base unit)
> 1 K is equal to 1/273.16 of the thermodynamic scale temperature of the triple point of water
> The Kelvin scale is an absolute thermodynamic temperature scale, using absolute zero as its null point.

Kilogram (kg): SI unit of mass (SI base unit)
> The standard kilogram is the mass of a cylindrical piece of platinum-iridium alloy kept in Sèvres, France.
> The only SI base unit with an SI prefix (Kilo)
> The only SI unit that is still defined by an artifact, and not a fundamental property that can be reproduced in a laboratory.

Kinetic energy:
> The energy a body possesses because of its motion
> It is defined as the energy needed to accelerate the object from a state of rest to its given velocity. This energy is equal to the work it would do when decelerating to return to rest.

Latent heat:
> The energy released or absorbed by a substance when it changes phase at a given temperature, e.g. ice melting
> The term 'latent' describes the 'hidden' change in energy state, as there is no change in the substance's temperature during this phase shift.

Latent heat of fusion (melting):
> The amount of heat required to convert a unit mass of a solid at its melting point into a liquid without an increase in temperature.

Latent heat of vaporisation:
> The amount of heat required to convert a unit mass of a liquid at its boiling point into vapour without an increase in temperature.

Mass:
> The amount of matter contained in a body
> The SI unit of mass = kilogram
> Unlike weight, mass does not alter under conditions of differing gravity.

Metre (m): SI unit of length (SI base unit)
> Originally defined as the length of a platinum-iridium bar kept near Paris, there were concerns about the bar's length changing over time.
> Since 1983, defined as the length of the path travelled by light in vacuum during the time interval of 1/299 792 458 of a second.

Mole: SI unit of amount of substance (SI base unit)
> Quantity containing the same number of particles as there are atoms in 12 g of carbon-12. This number of particles is 6.022×10^{23} and is known as Avogadro's constant.

Momentum:
> Mass × velocity

Newton (N): Derived SI unit of force
> 1 N is the force required to accelerate a mass of 1 kg by 1 m per second squared.

Ohm (Ω): Derived SI unit of electrical resistance
> 1 ohm is the resistance between two points of a conductor when a constant potential difference of 1 volt applied between them produces a current of 1 ampere.

Pascal (Pa): Derived SI unit of pressure
> 1 Pa is the force of 1 N acting over $1\,m^2$.

pH:
> The negative logarithm to the base 10 of the hydrogen ion concentration in a solution.
> $pH = -\log_{10}[H^+]$

Potential energy:
> The energy of a body or system as a result of its position in an electric, magnetic or gravitational field. It is the potential of that body to do work.

Power:
> The rate of doing work
> Unit of power = the watt
> 1 Watt = 1 joule per second

Pressure:
> Force per unit area
> Derived SI unit is the Pascal (Pa).

Relative humidity:
> The mass of water in a given volume of air, expressed as a percentage of the maximum mass of water that the air could hold at the given temperature.
> The ratio of the water vapour pressure to the saturated vapour pressure.

Resistance:
> Property of a conductor to oppose the flow of current through it.
> The derived SI unit of electrical resistance is the Ohm (Ω).

Saturated vapour pressure (SVP):
> The pressure exerted by a vapour when in contact with and in equilibrium with its liquid phase within a closed system at a given temperature.

Second (s): SI unit of time (SI base unit)
> Defined according to the frequency of radiation emitted by caesium-133 in its ground state.

Specific heat capacity (SHC):
> The amount of energy required to raise the temperature of 1 kg of a substance by 1 °C
> SHC of water = 4.16 kJ/kg °C
> SHC of human body = 3.5 kJ/kg °C.

Specific latent heat of vaporisation (boiling)
> The amount of heat required to convert a unit mass of a liquid at its boiling point into a gas without an increase in temperature, at a given pressure

Triple point of water:
> The temperature and pressure at which water exists in equilibrium as liquid water, solid ice and water vapour
> Temperature = 0.01 °C or 273.16 K, pressure = 0.006 atmosphere or 611.73 pascals.

Vapour:
> A substance in the gas phase below its critical temperature.

Volt (V): Derived SI unit of electrical potential
> 1 volt is the potential difference between two points of a conducting wire when 1 joule of work is done to move 1 coulomb of charge between them
> 1 volt is the potential difference between two points of a conducting wire when 1 ampere dissipates 1 watt of power between them
> 1 volt will 'push' a current of 1 ampere through a resistance of 1 Ohm.

Watt (W): Derived SI unit of power
> 1 watt = 1 joule per second.

Weight:
> The gravitational force acting on an object
> Measured in newtons
> Weight = mass in kg × gravitational acceleration ($9.81 \, ms^{-2}$). A mass of 1 kg will therefore have 9.81 N acting on it on the surface of the earth (and much less on the surface of the moon).

51. STANDARD INTERNATIONAL UNITS

The creation of the decimal metric system began during the eighteenth-century French revolution when two platinum standards, representing the metre and kilogram, were placed in the Archives de la République in Paris. Eminent scientists like Gauss and Weber then went on to promote the universal application of a standard system of measurement in the early nineteenth century. By the 1960s, the International System of Units (abbreviated to SI units from the French Le Système International d'Unités) was developed which incorporated six base units (the mole was added later) along with rules for the use of derived units and prefixes. The advantage of this unified system is that equations and calculations will produce answers in the appropriate SI unit. Unfortunately, they are not used universally.

A question concerning the SI units is a popular opening to the physics SOE and candidates should understand the relationship between derived and base units and be comfortable in manipulating them from one to the other.

What are the fundamental (base) units?

There are seven base units, which are considered to be dimensionally independent

Table 51.1   Base units

Base unit	Name	Symbol
Length	metre	m
Mass	kilogram	kg
Time	second	s
Current	ampere	A
Temperature	kelvin	K
Amount of substance	mole	mol
Luminous intensity	candela	cd

What are the two supplementary units?

The plane angle (radian) and solid angle (steradian) were supplementary units but this category was abolished in 1995. These units are considered named derived units.

List some of the derived units.

Derived units are formed by combination of various base units according to mathematical relationships which link these quantities.

Table 51.2 Derived units

Derived units	Name	Symbol
Area	square metre	m^2
Volume	cubic metre	m^3
Density	kilogram per cubic metre	kg/m^3
Velocity	metre per second	m/s
Acceleration	metre per second squared	m/s^2

List some named derived units.

These are derived units that have been given specific names.

Table 51.3 Named derived units

Named derived unit	Name (symbol)	Expression in terms of other SI units	Expression in terms of base SI units
Force	newton (N)	–	$kg \cdot m \cdot s^{-2}$
Pressure	pascal (Pa)	N/m^2	$kg \cdot m^{-1} \cdot s^{-2}$
Energy	joule (K)	$N \cdot m$	$kg \cdot m^2 \cdot s^{-2}$
Power	watt (W)	J/s	$kg \cdot m^2 \cdot s^{-3}$
Electric charge	coulomb (C)	–	$A \cdot s$
Electric potential difference	volt (V)	W/A	$kg \cdot m^2 \cdot s^{-3} \cdot A^{-1}$
Capacitance	farad (F)	C/V	$kg^{-1} \cdot m^{-2} \cdot s^4 \cdot A^2$
Electrical resistance	ohm (Ω)	V/A	$kg \cdot m^2 \cdot s^{-3} \cdot A^{-2}$
Magnetic flux	weber (Wb)	$V \cdot s$	$kg \cdot m^2 \cdot s^{-2} \cdot A^{-1}$
Magnetic flux density	tesla (T)	Wb/m^2	$kg \cdot s^{-2} \cdot A^{-1}$
Inductance	henry (H)	Wb/A	$kg \cdot m^2 \cdot s^{-2} \cdot A^{-2}$
Temperature	degree celsius (°C)	–	K

What are the common prefixes used for SI units?

Prefixes are decimal (base 10) multiples and submultiples of the quantity.

Table 51.4 Prefixes used for SI units

Prefix name (symbol)	Multiple	Prefix name (symbol)	Multiple
deca (da)	10^1	deci (d)	10^{-1}
hecto (h)	10^2	centi (c)	10^{-2}
kilo (k)	10^3	milli (m)	10^{-3}
mega (M)	10^6	micro (µ)	10^{-6}
giga (G)	10^9	nano (n)	10^{-9}
tera (T)	10^{12}	pico (p)	10^{-12}
peta (P)	10^{15}	femto (f)	10^{-15}
exa (E)	10^{18}	atto (a)	10^{-18}
zetta (Z)	10^{21}	zepto (z)	10^{-21}
yotta (Y)	10^{24}	yocto (y)	10^{-24}

52. PRINCIPLES OF MEASUREMENT

Describe the components of a standard measurement system.

Measurement systems are used to detect an input, transduce the signal and display it in a form that can be used by an interpreter.

They are made up of the following:

> **Input** – parameter chosen to be measured, e.g. blood pressure (BP).
> **Transducer** – device that converts one form of energy into another, e.g. the strain gauge inside an invasive BP monitoring transducer. The pressure generated by the arterial pulse alters the shape of the diaphragm on which strain gauges are arranged as a Wheatstone bridge. The deformation alters the length of the wire in the gauges and so their resistance is altered. The change in electrical signal is fed via the transmission path into the conditioning unit.
> **Transmission path** – apparatus that carries the electrical signal to the conditioning unit.
> **Conditioning unit** – apparatus in which the electrical signal is processed, analysed and then passed to the display unit.
> **Display unit** – monitor, gauge or dial on which the output is displayed.
> **Output** – final stage, and what is viewed on the screen, dial or gauge. The clinical context and the limitations of the equipment used must be taken into consideration when interpreting the output.

Measurement systems can either be **analogue** or **digital**.

> **Analogue** – output signal is continuous, e.g. the waveform display of an arterial pressure trace.
> **Digital** – output signal is discontinuous, e.g. the numerical display of BP next to the arterial waveform.

Which factors affect the output of a measurement system?

> **Accuracy** – this determines how closely the output reflects the true value being measured. Machines have their accuracy quoted as a percentage by the manufacturers, e.g. a machine that displayed 110 units when the true value was 100 would have an accuracy of ±10% across its working range.
> **Sensitivity** – this determines how small a change in input will result in a change in output. Less sensitive systems will be able to operate over a wider range.
> **Drift** – as the name suggests, this is a movement of the output away from the true input value. It is usually linear and unidirectional, although it does not have to be. It is usually caused by changing properties of the components of the equipment, e.g. ageing of thermistors.
> **Gain** – this refers to the degree of amplification of the measurement system (i.e. the output to input ratio).

What is hysteresis?

In a system with hysteresis, the output of the system alters depending on whether the input is rising or falling. In a system without hysteresis the output can be predicted from the input alone, but with hysteresis the operator needs to know the input history to estimate the output. An example of this is seen in the lung compliance curve, which exhibits hysteresis because of the elastic energy that is stored within it.

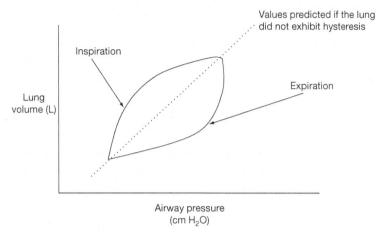

Fig. 52.1   Lung volume–pressure (compliance) curve showing hysteresis

What is damping?

This is definitely an answer to practise aloud before you go into the exam. Although it is intuitively simple to understand, damping can be surprisingly hard to explain. We think it is easiest to draw the next graph (Fig. 52.2) and use it to illustrate your answer.

Damping describes the resistance of a system to oscillation resulting from a change in the input. Damping is the result of frictional forces working in that system.

In the perfect measurement system, any change in input would be instantly and accurately reflected in the output. However, this is not the case in clinical systems and it takes time for a change in input to be reflected by a change in output. The speed with which this happens can be measured and defined:

> The '**response time**' is the time taken for the output to reach 90% of its final reading.
> The '**rise time**' is the time taken for the output to rise from 10 to 90% of its final reading.

Although it is impossible to design the 'perfect' system described above, we do need a system that responds as rapidly as possible to any change in input. This in itself can create problems, as a system that rises quickly will have the tendency to overshoot in its reading, while one which rises too slowly may never reach the new elevated input value, or may simply take too long to be a useful measure of a changing input.

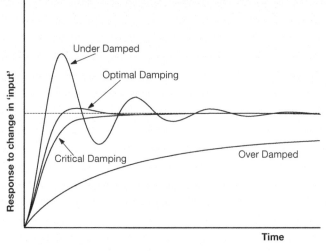

Fig. 52.2 Damping

So, following a change in input there are several possible outcomes for the system:

> **Perfect response** – described above.

> **Under-damped** – the output changes quickly in response to the step up in input, but it overshoots and then oscillates around the true value, before coming to rest at it. This means that it will be some time before the true value is displayed and the peaks and troughs will over- and under-represent the true value. In a dynamic system, e.g. intra-arterial BP, the constantly changing input may result in wild fluctuations, rendering an under-damped system very inaccurate (although the MAP is still correct).

> **Critically damped** – The response and rise time of the system are longer than an under-damped response, but there is no significant overshoot and oscillations are minimal. 'D' is the damping factor and, by convention, in a critically damped system **D = 1**.

> **Over-damped** – defined as damping greater than critical. The output here could potentially change so slowly that it never reaches the true value. In a dynamic system, the response time may be too slow for the system to be useful.

> **Optimally damped** – in reality in clinical measurement systems, critical damping is not ideal and we are prepared to accept a few oscillations and some overshoot to achieve a faster response time. Hence, our systems are '**optimally damped**' where 64% of the energy is removed from the system and **D = 0.64**. There is a 7% overshoot in this case.

What are the characteristics of the ideal invasive BP monitoring equipment?

> A short, stiff, wide cannula. This helps to keep its natural frequency high (*see* explanation of resonance and natural frequency below).

> No connections in the system, again to keep the natural frequency high.

> No air bubbles in the system as these are compressible and therefore decrease energy transmission up the column of fluid resulting in a damped trace.

What is calibration?

Calibration is a process in which the output of a measuring device is compared to a standard of known units of measure to determine the accuracy of the measuring device. For example, a blood gas machine may be primed with a solution of known pH and its output is compared with the known value of the solution. If the measuring device is proved to be inaccurate it can be reset accordingly.

Calibration should not be done against just one standard; at least two must be used. The more standards that are used for comparison, the more accurate will be the resultant measuring device.

Calibration should be performed when:

> A predetermined period of time has elapsed.
> The machine has been used a predetermined number of times.
> The machine gives unexpected results.
> The machine is moved, undergoes vibration or damage.

What is 'signal noise'?

Signal noise describes unwanted external information that is fed unintentionally into a transducer, resulting in the output being altered. We see this on the ECG display when diathermy is being used. Often here, the noise is so 'loud' that it actually obscures the ECG display. The magnitude of noise is described by comparing the two amplitudes to give the 'Signal:Noise (S/N) ratio'.

How can we overcome noise?

> We can add 'filters' into measurement systems, so that signals above or below given frequencies are 'ignored' and not processed to produce an output.
> • High pass filters ignore signals below a given frequency.
> • Low pass filters ignore signals above a given frequency.
> • Notch filters ignore signals at a given frequency, e.g. 50 Hz – mains frequency.

> We can average out the signal in cases where the signal is repetitive (as in most biological systems) and the noise is intermittent. This is useful when the noise is very loud compared to the desired signal.

RESONANCE AND NATURAL FREQUENCY

Resonance is the tendency of a system to oscillate at maximum amplitude at certain frequencies. This resonant frequency is determined by the mass and stiffness of the system. The greater the mass, the slower the oscillations, and the stiffer the system, the faster the oscillations.

The components of a measurement system will oscillate at their own natural frequency. Imagine that we are able to give energy to the system at the perfect moment to allow us to increase the amplitude of these oscillations. As the oscillations got bigger, it would be impossible to stop them being transmitted to the output reading. In this way, the *method* of measuring the true value would interfere with the output value displayed. For the 'physics challenged' among us, an easier way to visualise this is to imagine yourself on a swing. If you push off, and swing your legs at a steady rate, your swinging, or oscillation, will remain fairly constant. If, however, a friend comes and pushes you when you are at your highest point, they give energy to your system and you will swing higher and higher – your oscillations will increase in amplitude. If you were attached to an output monitor, you would see the units displayed increase. The key to this concept is that your friend has to push you at just the right point in your swing; too soon or too late, and they will not help increase your amplitude, and may even decrease it.

For our clinical example, think of the invasive BP transducer. If its natural frequency was near that of the input being measured (i.e. the swings up and down of the arterial pulse) it is easy to see how its own natural oscillations could be augmented by those of the pulse, which could act like the friend pushing the swing. The natural frequency of the arterial pulse is around 20 Hz (because it is comprised of lots of sine waves 'stacked' on top of each other, each with a frequency of approximately 2 Hz). For this reason, the manufacturers try to make the natural frequency of the transducer kit out of this range, and in fact most kits have a natural frequency of around 45 000 Hz.

This would work well, were it not for the way we then choose to use the carefully designed apparatus. We do not have the transducer in close proximity to the artery; instead we attach a long column of saline to the end of the transducer and attach this to the arterial cannula. This is for convenience, but it dramatically reduces the natural frequency of the measuring system. The long, heavy saline column reduces the natural frequency from 45 000 Hz to around 15 Hz and this brings the frequency of the measuring system very close to that of the input. Hence, it is now easy to see how the oscillations in BP can augment the oscillations of the measuring system and so give us falsely elevated and depressed peaks and troughs in our output display. This is the practical example of under-damping, when the arterial pressure is inappropriately over-represented.

At the beginning of the section on damping, we said that it was caused by friction in the measurement system. Using the example of being on the swing again, if you become frightened that your friend is pushing you too hard, and you are swinging too high, what do you do? You scrape your feet along the ground, increasing friction, dissipating energy and therefore reducing the amplitude of your oscillations.

The things that increase damping in our invasive BP monitoring system have been listed above. As users of the system, we cannot actually affect the natural frequency of the system. The only thing we can do theoretically is alter the length of the saline column, but even this is predetermined by the length of the tubing in the 'arterial line' packs. Increasing the length of the saline column will add to damping which you would think would be helpful given that we are worried about augmenting the system's natural oscillations. However, this will decrease the system's natural frequency to a more significant degree and so we tend to move towards an under-damped system, the longer the saline column.

53. GAS LAWS

As with most physics questions, the examiner is likely to start by asking you for definitions before trying to make the subject matter clinically relevant.

What is a gas?

A gas is a substance that exists above its critical temperature. This term is usually used colloquially to describe a substance whose critical temperature is below room temperature.

What is critical temperature (CT)?

This is the temperature above which a gas cannot be liquefied by the application of pressure alone (CT for O_2 is $-119\,°C$ and N_2O is $36.5\,°C$).

What is an 'ideal gas'?

An 'ideal gas' is a theoretical gas in which the molecules behave as individual particles that move in a random manner independent of each other and of any inter-molecular forces. At standard temperature and pressure (STP: 273.15 K and 101.3 kPa) most gases behave qualitatively like an ideal gas. The 'ideal gas' is a useful concept because it obeys the ideal gas laws.

What are the gas laws?

The gas laws are a set of rules that govern the relationship between thermodynamic temperature, volume and pressure of ideal gases.

> **Boyle's law:** At a constant temperature, the absolute pressure of a given mass of gas is inversely proportional to the volume.

(density = mass/volume $\rightarrow$ density $\propto$ 1/volume $\rightarrow$ pressure $\propto$ density)

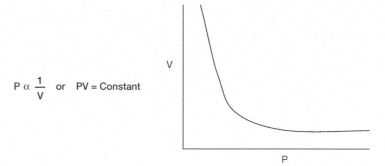

$$P \alpha \frac{1}{V} \quad \text{or} \quad PV = \text{Constant}$$

Fig. 53.1 Boyle's law

> **Charles's law:** At a constant pressure, the volume of a given mass of gas is directly proportional to the absolute temperature.

$V \propto T$ or $\dfrac{V}{T}$ = Constant

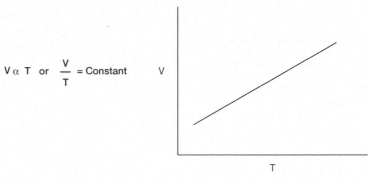

Fig. 53.2 Charles's law

> **Gay-Lussac's law:** At a constant volume, the absolute pressure of a given mass of gas varies directly with the absolute temperature. This is also known as the third perfect gas law.

$P \propto T$ or $\dfrac{P}{T}$ = Constant

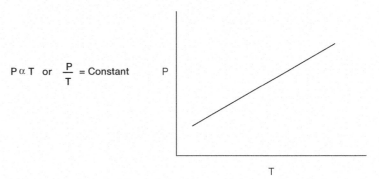

Fig. 53.3 Gay-Lussac's law

> All of these laws have been united into one, **the Ideal Gas Equation**, which comes from the premise that in an ideal gas, a given number of particles will occupy the same volume at a given temperature and pressure.

$$\frac{PV}{T} = \text{Constant}$$

> Using this equation, it is possible to convert one set of conditions to another because for a given mass of gas:

$$\frac{P_1 V_1}{T_1} = \frac{P_2 V_2}{T_2}$$

> The ideal gas equation is usually written as:

$$PV = nRT$$

Where:
n = number of moles of gas present
R = universal gas constant = 8.32144 J/K/mol

What is Avogadro's hypothesis?	> This states that equal volumes of gases at a given temperature and pressure contain the same numbers of molecules. > One mole of a gas at STP will occupy 22.4 L and will contain 6.022×10^{23} particles (Avogadro's number).
What is Avogadro's number?	> One mole of a substance contains the same number of particles as there are atoms in 12 g of carbon-12 (i.e. 6.022×10^{23}). > This number of particles is known as Avogadro's number.

Give an example where we may use Avogadro's hypothesis

Avogadro's hypothesis is used to calculate the contents of a N_2O cylinder:

$$\text{No. of moles of } N_2O \text{ in cylinder} = \frac{\text{Weight of } N_2O}{\text{Molecular weight of } N_2O}$$

$$= \frac{\text{(Cylinder weight – Tare weight)}}{44}$$

$$\text{Volume of } N_2O \text{ available (L)} = \text{No. of moles} \times 22.4\,L$$

What are the clinical applications of these gas laws?

The ideal gas law ($P_1V_1/T_1 = P_2V_2/T_2$) is used to calculate the volume of O_2 available from an O_2 cylinder:

> Cylinder capacity is fixed = 10 L [V_1]
> Gauge pressure of cylinder = 13 700 kP$_a$
> Absolute pressure of cylinder = gauge pressure (13 700 kP$_a$) + atmospheric pressure (100 kP$_a$) = 13 800 kP$_a$ [P_1]
> Volume of O_2 available = [V_2]
> Absolute pressure of atmosphere = 100 kP$_a$ [P_2]
> As temperature is constant, $T_1 = T_2$ and hence equation is further simplified

$$P_1 \times V_1 = P_2 \times V_2 \rightarrow 13\,800 \times 10 = 100 \times V_2 \rightarrow V_2 = 1380\,L$$

> But 10 L will always remain in the cylinder, and hence 1370 L of O_2 is available.

An alternative approach to this is to use the ideal gas law ($PV/T = nRT$) to calculate the contents of a gas cylinder:
> Volume of the cylinder is fixed
> R is a constant
> Temperature is fixed
> Therefore, pressure is directly related to the number of moles of gas (which can be converted into a volume using Avogadro's hypothesis).

The ideal gas law is used in the adiabatic process:

> If heat energy is not added to or lost from a system, a rapid compression of gas will result in a rise in its temperature, and conversely a sudden expansion will result in a fall.
> This principle is harnessed by the cryotherapy probe used to freeze lesions in surgery where a sudden expansion of gas through the end leaves its tip extremely cold.

What is Dalton's law of partial pressures?

This states that the total pressure exerted by a gaseous mixture is equal to the sum of the partial pressures of each of the individual gases within that mixture.

What is Henry's law?

This states that the amount of gas dissolved in a liquid is proportional to its partial pressure above that liquid at a given temperature (the warmer the liquid, the less gas that dissolves in it, and that is why boiling water bubbles because air comes out of the liquid phase).

54. SUPPLY OF MEDICAL GASES

How is oxygen manufactured?

> The most common method of manufacturing oxygen commercially is by the fractional distillation of liquefied air. This method produces oxygen which is over 99% pure.
> Alternatively, oxygen concentrators containing zeolite adsorbents can be used. Zeolite selectively adsorbs nitrogen and so delivers oxygen that is 90–93% pure. The major contaminant is argon. Oxygen concentrators are commonly used in aircraft, submarines, military field hospitals and at home.

How is oxygen stored?

> The main hospital supply of oxygen comes from a vacuum-insulated evaporator (VIE), which holds up to 1500 L of liquid oxygen. This is the most economical and space-saving way of storing oxygen. The liquid oxygen is stored at a temperature between –150 and –170 °C (below its critical temperature of –119 °C) and at a pressure of 7 bar (this is the saturated vapour pressure (SVP) of oxygen at its stored temperature). Because it is in liquid form, oxygen in a VIE behaves like nitrous oxide in a cylinder and therefore in order to know how much oxygen is remaining, the storage vessel rests on a weighing balance so that the mass of liquid oxygen can be measured.
> The hospital back-up oxygen supply comes from a cylinder manifold (size J cylinders arranged in series), which stores oxygen as a compressed gas at room temperature. The oxygen from these sites gets carried to the hospital in pipelines coloured white delivered at a pressure of 4 bar (400 kP$_a$).
> Oxygen on the anaesthetic machine is stored as a compressed gas in molybdenum steel cylinders (size E cylinders) with black bodies and white shoulders at a pressure of 137 bar (13 700 kP$_a$).

Why are oxygen cylinders filled to 137 bar?

Cylinder technology is old and filling pressures of compressed gases were originally measured in pounds per square inch (psi). The cylinders were filled to 2000 psi, which is equivalent to 137 bar.

How do you calculate the volume of oxygen that can be discharged from a 10 L cylinder?

Oxygen in a cylinder is stored as a compressed gas and obeys the ideal gas law ($P_1V_1/T_1 = P_2V_2/T_2$), which is used to calculate the volume of O$_2$ available:

> Cylinder capacity is fixed = 10 L [V_1]
> Gauge pressure of cylinder = 13 700 kP$_a$
> Absolute pressure of cylinder = gauge pressure (13 700 kP$_a$) + atmospheric pressure (100 kP$_a$) = 13 800 kP$_a$ [P_1]
> Volume of O$_2$ available = [V_2]
> Pressure of atmosphere = 100 kP$_a$ [P_2]

> As temperature is constant, $T_1 = T_2$ and hence equation is further simplified

$$P_1 \times V_1 = P_2 \times V_2 \rightarrow 13\,800 \times 10 = 100 \times V_2 \rightarrow V_2 = 1380\,L$$

> But 10 L will always remain in the cylinder, and hence 1370 L of O_2 is available.

Draw a graph showing what would happen to the gauge pressure of an oxygen cylinder over time if it were being used continuously at the same rate

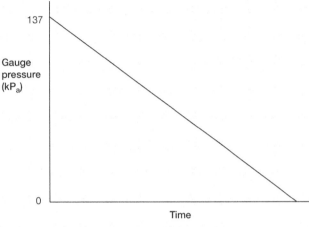

Fig. 54.1 Change in gauge pressure over time for an O_2 cylinder

How is nitrous oxide manufactured?

Nitrous oxide (N_2O) is manufactured by the thermal decomposition of ammonium nitrate.

How is nitrous oxide stored?

> The critical temperature of nitrous oxide is 36.5 °C and therefore at room temperature N_2O exists as a liquid with its vapour.
> On the anaesthetic machine, N_2O is stored as a liquid in molybdenum steel cylinders with blue bodies and blue shoulders at a pressure of 52 bar (this is the SVP of N_2O vapour above its liquid).
> N_2O cylinders are only partially filled because liquids are less compressible than gases and should these cylinders be subjected to temperatures above its critical temperature (e.g. in a desert or during a fire) all the N_2O would convert to a gas, causing a massive explosion. Therefore, depending on the temperature of the country, N_2O cylinders have different filling ratios.

$$\textbf{The filling ratio} \; = \; \frac{\textbf{Weight of substance cylinder is routinely filled with}}{\textbf{Weight of water cylinder could hold if full}}$$

> In tropical countries the filling ratio is 0.67 but in temperate climates it is 0.75.
> The main hospital supply of N_2O comes from a cylinder manifold where once again the N_2O is stored as a liquid at room temperature.

Why do different textbooks quote varying gauge pressures for N_2O cylinders?

N_2O cylinder gauge pressures reflect the SVP of the N_2O above its liquid and are quoted from between 44 and 54 bar depending on the temperature at which the measurement was taken (as SVP varies with temperature).

How can you calculate the volume of N₂O that can be discharged from a cylinder?

Because these cylinders contain liquid and vapour you cannot apply the ideal gas law. Instead you need to weigh the cylinder in order to work out the weight of the remaining N_2O and then apply Avogadro's hypothesis:

$$\text{No. of moles of } N_2O \text{ in cylinder} = \frac{\text{Weight of } N_2O}{\text{Molecular weight of } N_2O}$$

$$= \frac{(\text{Cylinder weight} - \text{Tare weight})}{44}$$

Volume of N_2O available (L) = No. of moles × 22.4 L

Avogadro's hypothesis states that at standard temperature and pressure 1 mole of gas occupies 22.4 L.

Draw a graph showing what would happen to the gauge pressure of a nitrous oxide cylinder over time if it were being used continuously at the same rate

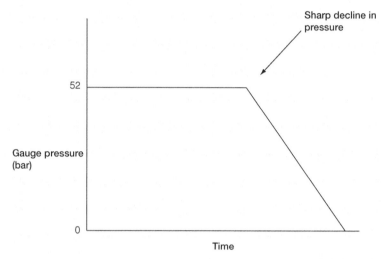

Fig. 54.2 Change in gauge pressure over time for a N_2O cylinder

> Initially, the N_2O cylinder contains both liquid and vapour.
> As the cylinder empties, the vapour is used up and the liquid continues to vaporise until it is all used up.
> This explains the constant cylinder gauge pressure until all the liquid has been used up, at which point the cylinder only contains gas and behaves like the oxygen cylinder and obeys Boyle's law, with pressure declining over time with use.
> This is actually a simplification; in reality the initial pressure is not perfectly constant because as the N_2O vaporises from the liquid phase it cools slightly (latent heat of vaporisation), and therefore gauge pressure does fall slightly.

Define the following terms.

> **Gas** – substance which is above its critical temperature. A gas will expand to fill any space available.
> **Vapour** – a gas below its critical temperature.
> **Critical temperature** – temperature above which a substance cannot be liquefied no matter how much pressure is applied.
> **Pseudocritical temperature** – applies to a mixture of gases (e.g. entonox; 50% O_2 and 50% N_2O) and is the temperature at which these gases may separate out into their individual constituents.
> **Critical pressure** – pressure required to liquefy a gas at its critical temperature.

What is the Poynting effect?

If a gas mixture is exposed to a temperature below its pseudocritical temperature the individual gas components can liquefy and separate out. This is known as the Poynting effect and is important in relation to entonox cylinders. If entonox cylinders are allowed to fall below −5.5 °C (e.g. during mountain rescues) a liquid mixture containing mostly N_2O with only about 20% O_2 dissolved in it can form along with a high oxygen content gas mixture just above it. If this cylinder is then used, the patient will initially receive an O_2-rich gas mixture but as the cylinder is used up the O_2 concentration will progressively decrease and eventually the patient may receive a hypoxic gas mixture. In order to minimise these risks, entonox cylinders should be stored horizontally at temperatures above 5 °C.

Table 54.1 Key features of commonly used medical gases

Content	State	Cylinder colour (cylinder/shoulder)	Cylinder pressure (bar)	Critical temperature (°C)
Oxygen	Gas	Black/White	137	−119
Nitrous oxide	Vapour	Blue/Blue	52	36.5
Air	Gas	Black/Black & White	137	−141
Carbon dioxide	Vapour	Grey/Grey	50	31
Entonox	Gas mix	Blue/Blue & White	137	−5.5 (pseudocritical)
Heliox	Gas	Brown/Brown & White	137	

55. GENERAL ASPECTS OF PRESSURE

'Dum dum dum didi da dum insanity laughs under pressure we're cracking'

— David Bowie

Questions on pressure can start innocently enough but can lead to almost any aspect of anaesthesia. One college question starts by comparing the pressure generated in 2 and 20 mL syringes and ends up with altitude effects via calibration of pressure transducers.

Define pressure.

Pressure is the force applied per unit area. Its SI unit is the pascal (N/m^2).

What is force?

Force is a vector quantity that can cause an object with mass to accelerate. Newton's second law defined force as the mass of an object multiplied by its acceleration. Its SI unit is the newton.

One newton will accelerate a 1 kg mass at $1 \, m/s^2$ in a vacuum. Gravity gives any object an acceleration of $9.81 \, m/s^2$ making one newton equivalent to a 102 g weight. This is a small pressure when applied to a squared metre area, so pressure is normally expressed in kilopascals (kP_a).

What other units of pressure are there?

1 bar is equivalent to:

> 1 atmosphere
> 14.5 lb/in^2 (psi)
> 30 inches of Hg
> 101 kP_a
> 760 mmHg (torr)
> 1020 cm H_2O

Are you more likely to dislodge a blockage in a cannula when using a 2 or 20 mL syringe?

A 2 mL syringe, as pressure is force over area. The 2 mL syringe has a smaller cross-sectional area so the force applied by the thumb is spread over a smaller area generating a higher pressure. For this reason care must be taken when injecting fluids with a small syringe as the high pressure generated could cause tissue damage.

What is the difference between partial and total pressures?

Dalton's law states that in a gas mixture the pressure exerted by each individual gas is equal to the pressure that gas would exert if it occupied the container alone. This is the partial pressure (the term 'tension' refers to the pressure exerted by a gas dissolved in liquid). Total pressure is the sum of all the partial pressures in the mixture.

Is atmospheric pressure constant?

No. Atmospheric pressure is created by the force of gravity acting on the molecules that make up the atmosphere and therefore atmospheric pressure will depend on the height of the atmosphere and its density. This means that atmospheric pressure will fall with altitude and rising temperature. As a consequence, the partial pressure of the gases that make up the air will also fall, leading to low partial pressures of oxygen at altitude.

What is gauge pressure?

Gauge pressure refers to pressure measurements above or below atmospheric pressure. An empty cylinder pressure will have a gauge pressure of zero.

What is absolute pressure?

Absolute pressure refers to pressure measurements incorporating atmospheric pressure – it is gauge pressure plus atmospheric pressure. An empty cylinder will have an absolute pressure of 1 bar.

Is blood pressure an absolute or gauge pressure?

Blood pressure is a gauge pressure.

How do manometers work?

> A manometer consists of a fluid-filled column, which is open to the atmosphere and therefore reads gauge pressure.
> Gravity acts on the fluid to produce a pressure, which is dependent on the density of the fluid and the height of the fluid but independent of the cross-sectional area of the column (pressure = height × density × gravitational force).
> They are used to measure low pressures.
> Inaccuracies can be caused by surface tension. This leads to an over-reading in water manometers and an under-reading in mercury manometers (in practice this has no clinical significance as a 6-mm-wide column of water will only over-read by $0.04\,kP_a$).
> They can be made more sensitive by using fluids with a low density (e.g. a pressure of $1\,kP_a$ will support a column of mercury 7.5 mm high or a column of water 10.2 cm high).

What are barometers?

> Barometers are closed to the atmosphere and therefore measure absolute pressure.
> A mercury barometer has a Torricellian vacuum above it, which contains mercury vapour at its saturated vapour pressure (SVP).
> Barometers like the Fortin's barometer and Goethe's device can be used to measure sub-atmospheric pressures. Here, the height of the measuring column falls rather than rising and this principle was used to predict bad weather; low atmospheric pressures would cause a fall in the height of the fluid in a 'thunder tube', predicting an oncoming storm.

How do aneroid gauges work?

> Aneroid gauges (from the Greek meaning 'no water') such as the Bourdon gauge are used to measure high pressures where manometers would be impractical (e.g. to measure the pressure of a 137 bar oxygen cylinder you would need a mercury column 104 m high or a water column 1394 m high!).
> A Bourdon gauge consists of a coiled metal tube linked to a cog and a pointer. The cross-sectional area of the tube is elliptical and when exposed to increases in pressure it changes to a circular cross-sectional shape, which causes the tube to uncoil, moving the pointer across a scale.

56. PRESSURE REGULATORS

Questions about pressure regulators are likely to start with simple quick questions about the different pressures that gases are stored and delivered at and then move on to how these changes in pressure are achieved.

What are the pressures at which the common anaesthetic gases are stored and delivered at?

Table 56.1 Storage and delivery pressures for commonly used medical gases

Site	Oxygen	Air	Nitrous oxide
Cylinder pressure	137 bar	137 bar	52 bar (room temp.)
Pipeline pressure	4 bar	4 bar	4 bar
Common gas outlet pressure	2 cm H_2O	2 cm H_2O	2 cm H_2O

Define the following terms.

Pressure – force per unit area. The SI unit is the pascal (N/m^2). Other commonly used units are the kilopascal, mmHg, cm H_2O, psi, bar, torr and atm (*see* Chapter 55, 'General aspects of pressure').
Pressure regulators (or pressure-reducing valves) – devices that reduce a higher variable inlet pressure to a constant lower outlet pressure.

What different types of pressure regulators do you know?

The different types of pressure regulators may be classified as follows:

> **Direct** – where the cylinder pressure opens the valve
> **Indirect** – where a spring opens the valve in response to falling outlet pressure
> **Two-stage** – where the input of one is the output of the other, this reduces wear on the diaphragm and reduces pressure fluctuations in high gas flows (e.g. demand valves used on entonox cylinders)
> **Slave** – where the output of one valve is dependent on the output of another (e.g. nitrous oxide valve will not open unless there is output from the O_2 valve).

Why is the gas cylinder on an anaesthetic machine not connected directly to the rotameter block?

Gas (and vapour) cylinders are used to store gases and vapours at high pressures. These pressures vary according to the type of gas or vapour used, the cylinder content and temperature. The temperature and cylinder content will in turn vary as the gas or vapour is used. If unregulated this would lead to a variable flow of gas or vapour to the patient. In order to provide a safe and constant mixture of gases during anaesthesia, it is important to protect both the patient and anaesthetic machine from exposure to higher pressures, surges in pressure when cylinders are opened and changes in flow. This is achieved by using pressure regulators, flow restrictors and pressure relief valves. It is important to note that the pressure regulators are specific to particular gases and are set during servicing.

How does a single-stage regulator work?

> Pressure regulators consist of two chambers, a high-pressure chamber and a low or control pressure chamber, separated by a conical valve whose orifice is controlled by a spring connected to a diaphragm in the control chamber.
> They work by balancing the force from the spring against the force generated by pressure against the diaphragm.
> This shows that the performance of the valve is related to the ratio of the areas of the diaphragm and the valve: the bigger the difference, the greater the drop in pressure for the same force applied by the spring.

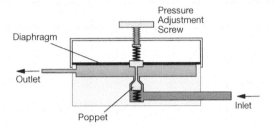

Fig. 56.1   Single-stage pressure regulator

> From the diagram it can be seen that if the inlet pressure (P) increases, the diaphragm will lift and the conical valve will shut and vice versa. The pressure in the control chamber can be fixed or varied by altering the tension in the spring.

How does a two-stage pressure regulator work?

> A demand valve on an entonox cylinder or diving cylinder is an example of a two-stage pressure regulator.
> The first stage of the regulator is identical to that already described, but now the flow of gas from the low-pressure chamber enters the second-stage chamber.
> The second-stage chamber contains a larger diaphragm that operates a valve, which connects it to the first-stage low-pressure chamber.
> The demand valve detects when the patient inspires and supplies a breath of gas at ambient pressure.
> As the patient inspires, the pressure within the second-stage chamber reduces, moving the diaphragm, which opens the valve and allows gas to enter the second-stage chamber from the first-stage low-pressure chamber.

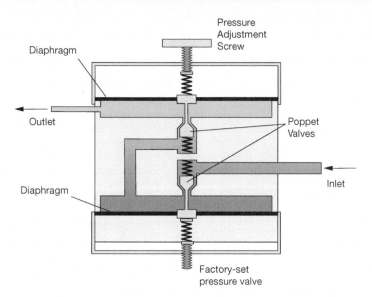

Fig. 56.2 Two-stage pressure regulator

How does the Ritchie whistle work?

> The Ritchie whistle is an oxygen failure alarm which is powered solely by falling oxygen pressures.
> It was invented by John Ritchie, a New Zealand anaesthetist, and was introduced into practice in the mid-1960s.
> Again, its design was tailored around a single-stage pressure regulator.
> Its working principle is simple: as the oxygen pressure falls, the force acting on the diaphragm reduces and a point is reached when the opposing force applied by the spring is greater, allowing the valve to open and oxygen to leak past and activate the whistle.
> Current oxygen failure devices must have an auditory sound of at least 60 dB lasting for 7 seconds and should be activated when oxygen pressure falls to $200 \, kP_a$. It should be linked to a system that shuts off the supply of all other gases apart from oxygen and air.
> Modern devices now use electronic sensors.

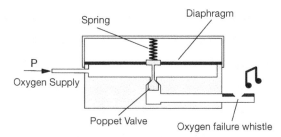

Fig. 56.3 Ritchie whistle

57. FLOW

A number of different liquids and gases are given to patients during a routine anaesthetic and, therefore, the physical properties of flow are essential to our practice. Examination questions can therefore take various directions (e.g. fluid administration though cannula, ventilating though different-sized endotracheal tubes, physics of rotameters and use of heliox). However, the fundamental principles regarding flow are the same irrespective of the application.

What is flow?

> Flow (F) is the quantity (Q) of a liquid or gas passing a point per unit time (t).
> A simplified equation for this is: $F = Q/t$.
> There are two main types of flow – laminar and turbulent flow, both of which have very different physical characteristics.

What are the characteristics of laminar flow?

> Fluid moves in a steady manner (no eddies or turbulence).
> Flow rate is greatest at the centre of the flow stream (2 × flow rate at side of tube).
> A pressure difference must exist for fluid to flow.
> Flow is directly proportional to this pressure difference.
> Resistance of the tube is calculated by the ratio of pressure to flow.

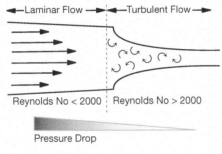

Fig. 57.1 Laminar and turbulent flow

What equation can be used to calculate laminar flow?

Hagen–Poiseuille equation is used to calculate laminar flow:

$$Flow = \frac{\pi \times \Delta P \times r^4}{8 \times L \times n}$$

Where:

π = Pi (mathematical constant – the ratio of any circle's circumference to its diameter)
ΔP = Pressure drop
r = Radius
L = Length of tube
n = Viscosity of fluid

Thus:

> Flow is proportional to the pressure drop and radius to the power of 4 of the tube.
> Flow is inversely proportional to the length of tube and the viscosity of the fluid.

Give an example where the Hagen–Poiseuille equation is clinically applied.	Administering a unit of blood rapidly to a patient:

Administering a unit of blood rapidly to a patient:

> Use a short, wide-bore cannula (i.e. a 16 G short cannula is better than using the 16 G distal port of a long central line)
> Raise the height of the giving set.
> Apply a pressure bag to the unit of blood.
> Warm the blood (reduces viscosity).

What are the characteristics of turbulent flow?

> Flow characterised by swirls and eddies.
> Transition of laminar to turbulent flow may occur at constrictions.
> Fluid velocity varies across the tube.
> Flow is proportional to the square root of pressure (i.e. to double flow, the pressure must be increased by a factor of 4).
> Resistance is no longer constant because the relationship between pressure and flow is no longer linear.
> Density of the fluid is the important determinant in turbulent flow (as opposed to fluid viscosity in laminar flow).

Thus:
> Flow is proportional to the square root of pressure.
> Flow is proportional to the radius squared.
> Flow is inversely proportional to the square root of the tube length.
> Flow is inversely proportional to the square root of fluid density.

What is Reynolds number?

This is a number that predicts the onset of turbulent flow of a fluid:

$$\text{Reynolds number} = \frac{\text{Velocity of fluid} \times \text{Density} \times \text{Tube diameter}}{\text{Viscosity}}$$

> Reynolds number < 2000 predicts laminar flow.
> Reynolds number > 2000 predicts turbulent flow.

(NB: Reynolds number does not have any units – it is a dimensionless number.)

Give an example where the concept of Reynolds number is used clinically.

Heliox is a mixture of 21% oxygen and 79% helium. Helium is much less dense than nitrogen, making heliox much less dense than air (about three times less dense). This reduction in density lowers the Reynolds number, which changes turbulent flow to laminar flow. Laminar flow is known to reduce the work of breathing.

What is the critical velocity?

This is the velocity above which the flow of a fluid within a given tube is likely to change from laminar to turbulent (e.g. critical velocity of gas flow in a 9 mm endotracheal tube is 9 L/min).

What is the Bernoulli principle?

In fluid dynamics, the Bernoulli principle refers to a lowering of fluid pressure in regions where the flow velocity increased. At a constriction point within a tube, the kinetic energy of a fluid increases and due to the 'law of conservation of energy' this means that the potential energy associated with its pressure at this point must fall in order for the total energy to remain constant.

What is the Venturi principle?

This uses the Bernoulli effect – the pressure drop induced by the increase in velocity of a fluid through a narrow orifice is used to entrain a second fluid at this point of low pressure. The **entrainment ratio** describes the ratio of entrained flow to driving flow. The Venturi principle is used in oxygen-enrichment face masks (e.g. venturi face masks), nebulisers, suction devices, scavenging systems and also to test the Bain circuit on the anaesthetic machine.

What is the Coandă effect?

This is the tendency of a fluid jet to stay attached to an adjacent curved surface. The principle was named after Henry Coandă, who was the first to recognise the practical application of the phenomenon in the development of jet engines. This tendency of fluid flow to not divide evenly explains the maldistribution of gas flow to alveoli where there has been a slight narrowing of the bronchiole before it divides.

How can flow be measured?

> **Wright respirometer:** This device actually measures gas volumes but flow can be calculated by measuring the volume of gas per unit time.
> - Device used to measure tidal volumes in anaesthesia.
> - Gas flow rotates vanes
> - Inaccurate for continuous flow
> - Over-reads at high flow rates
> - Under-reads at low flow rates

> **Pneumotachograph:** A constant orifice, variable-pressure device used to measure flow.
> - Flow is calculated by measuring the pressure difference across a fixed orifice.
> - Device used to measure gas flow.
> - A constant orifice, variable pressure device.
> - Gauze screen acts as a resistance to flow and maintains laminar flow.
> - Airflow causes a pressure drop across the gauze screen, which is measured by a pressure transducer and correlates with flow.
> - Pressure difference across the gauze is proportional to flow (provided flow is laminar).
> - Pressure change is converted into an electrical signal and displayed.

> **Rotameter:** A constant pressure, variable orifice device used in anaesthetic machines to act as a continuous indicator of gas flows.
> - Device used to measure gas flow.
> - Constant pressure, variable orifice device.
> - Bobbin in a tapered glass tube.
> - Rotating bobbin rises as flow increases.
> - Pressure across the bobbin remains constant.
> - Mixture of laminar and turbulent flow exists, therefore for calibration purposes, both the viscosity and density of the fluid are important.
> - Electrostatic charges can develop around the bobbin, which is minimised by the incorporation of a conductive strip.

What do you understand by the term 'fluidics'?

Fluidics is the technology of using the flow characteristics of a liquid or gas to perform analogue or digital operations similar to those performed by mechanical or electronic systems.

58. ELECTRICAL COMPONENTS

Questions on electrical components are often asked as part of a question on defibrillators (see Chapter 59, 'Defibrillators'). Typically, a card with various electrical symbols will be shown to the candidate, and this will lead on to questions regarding the various components. Another favourite topic is amplification and the Wheatstone bridge, including the concept of null deflection, so it is worth spending the time to understand how these work.

Explain the following terms.

> **Resistance:**
  - Is the opposition to flow of direct current.
  - It is represented by the symbols R and its unit is the ohm (Ω).
  - $1\,\Omega$ is the resistance that will allow 1 A of current to flow when a potential of 1 V is applied across it.
  - The resistance of different electrical components can vary with physical stresses such as temperature and stretch. These changes are exploited in electrical thermometers and transducers.
  - Resistance is key to Ohm's law ($V = I \times R$), which is a fundamental equation in electronics.

> **Reactance:**
  - Is the opposition to the flow of alternating current caused by the inductance and capacitance in a circuit rather than by resistance.
  - Capacitative reactance decreases with increasing frequency.
  - Inductive reactance increases with increasing frequency.
  - It is represented by the symbol X and its unit is the Ω.

> **Impedance:**
  - Total opposition to current flow in an alternating current circuit, made up of two components, resistance and reactance.
  - It is represented by the symbol Z and its unit is the Ω.

> **Capacitor:**
  - A device that can store charge.
  - It consists of two conducting plates separated by an insulator (dielectric).
  - The amount of charge that it can store depends on the size of the plates, separation gap and the dielectric material.
  - It blocks DC (high resistance) but passes AC (low reactance) as the plates get alternately charged and discharged.
  - As capacitative reactance decreases with increasing current frequency, diathermy devices with high frequencies of 1.5 MHz will have low reactance and hence will be conducted. Mains electricity at 50 Hz has a high reactance and therefore will not be conducted. This property makes capacitors useful filters.

- The capacitor's stored energy can also be discharged rapidly, making it the central component of the defibrillator.
- Charge (Q) is measured in coulombs (C), 1 C being the number of electrons passing a point when a current of 1 A flows for 1 s (6.24×10^{18} electrons).
- Capacitance (C) is measured in farads (F), 1 F being the capacity to hold 1 C of charge when a potential difference of 1 V is applied.
- The energy stored by a capacitor is given by the formula $E = \frac{1}{2}QV$ or $E = \frac{1}{2}CV^2$.

> **Inductor:**
  - A device that resists a change in electric current.
  - It consists of a wire coiled around a ferrous core (former).
  - As current flows through the coiled wire a magnetic field is generated.
  - These block AC (high reactance) but pass DC (low resistance).
  - These are a source of interference in electrical equipment where electromotive activity in one circuit can induce unwanted signals in another.
  - They are used in transformers and to isolate equipment from earth (floating circuits – *see* Chapter 60, 'Electrical safety') and are also used in defibrillators to smooth and lengthen the current pulse.

> **Transformer:**
  - A device which transfers electrical energy between two or more circuits through electro-magnetic induction.
  - They are used to increase (step up) or decrease (step down) the voltages of alternative current in electrical applications.
  - They consist of two inductors wound around the same former (core). This close relationship means that current changes in one circuit can induce current in the second circuit due to the coupling effects of the magnetic field.
  - They are used to step up the voltage of a current to allow efficient transmission over large distances and to step the voltage down to levels suitable for household use.
  - They are also used as isolating transformers (*see* Chapter 60, 'Electrical Safety') where they isolate appliances from earth.
  - The change in voltage from the primary circuit to the secondary circuit is calculated from Faraday's law of induction, where the ratio of the number of coils of each circuit around the transformer core determines whether there is an increase or decrease in the voltage from one to the other.

> **Earth:**
  - A system of electrical safety where there is an electrical connection to ground.
  - This protects people from the effects of faulty insulation in electrically powered equipment, as there is significantly less resistance through the earth circuit than there is through the person, and so electricity will flow preferentially through the former.
  - Class 1 equipment is earthed (*see* Chapter 60, 'Electrical Safety').

> **Diode (or rectifier):**
  - Allows current to flow in one direction only.

> **Battery (galvanic or voltaic cell):**
>   • A collection of galvanic cells that convert stored chemical energy into electrical energy when part of an electrical circuit.
>   • They consist of two half-cells (positive anode and negative cathode) connected by a conductive electrolyte.
>   • Oxidation occurs at the anode and reduction at the cathode, allowing a flow of electrons between the two.

> **Transducer:**
>   • A device which changes one form of energy into another, normally into an electronic signal for interpretation and recording.
>   • Examples include the microphone, which converts sound energy into an electrical signal, and the pressure transducer, which converts pressure changes into electrical resistance.

> **Amplifier:**
>   • This differs from a transducer in that it makes the input signal larger for easier interpretation rather than changing it from one form to another.
>   • They are used because biological signals are often very small (EEG signals in the order of micro-volts) and need to be made bigger (amplified) for display.
>   • Amplifiers do not need to be electrical. Levers can produce a large movement at one end of a needle from a small movement at the other (Bourdon gauge) and microscopes convert a small light field into a large one.
>   • For electrical signals, amplifiers increase the amplitude of the signal.
>   • The difference in the size of the input signal and the amplified signal is called the gain and is measured in bels (or decibels).
>   • In the amplification process there will inevitably be an amplification of unwanted signal. This is called the noise. The amount of noise introduced compared to the signal is called the signal to noise ratio and is a measure of the performance of the system.
>   • To reduce the amount of noise, amplifiers can also act as filters. They can achieve this in a number of ways. First, amplifiers are often differential amplifiers (also called operational amplifiers), that is they look for signals that vary from one source to another (e.g. different leads on an ECG) and amplify them, rejecting signals that are common to both as interference. This is called common mode rejection. If we consider the ECG signal again, the R wave will differ from lead to lead and so will be amplified for the ECG trace. However, 50 Hz mains interference will be the same at all leads and so will be rejected. Amplifiers also filter by amplifying only a certain frequency range (bandwidth filter), signals above or below a certain frequency (high or low pass filters), rejecting particular frequencies (notch filter, e.g. 50 Hz mains signal) and by amplifying signals of a particular amplitude.

59. DEFIBRILLATORS

Defibrillators are devices used to restore normal cardiac rhythm by delivering a burst of electrical energy to the heart. This 'burst' depolarises all the myocytes essentially re-setting the electrical status of the heart and allowing co-ordinated myocardial depolarisation to occur again. There are various types that can be manual or automated, monophasic or biphasic, external, transvenous or implanted in the patient.

What is the difference between monophasic and biphasic waveform defibrillators?

> **Monophasic waveform:** This is a damped sinusoidal wave (Lown-type waveform). Current flows in one direction only, from one electrode to the other.

> **Biphasic waveform:** This can be either a biphasic truncated exponential waveform or a rectilinear biphasic waveform. Current flows in alternating directions, completing one cycle in approximately 10 ms. During the first phase, current flows in one direction and then reverses direction during the second phase. This lowers the electrical threshold for successful defibrillation, allowing lower energy levels to be used and reducing the risk of burns and myocardial damage. Biphasic defibrillation was originally developed and used for implantable cardioverter defibrillators.

Draw the major components in a defibrillator circuit.

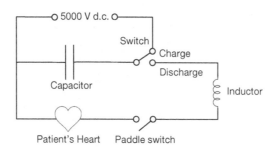

Fig. 59.1 Components of a defibrillator circuit

How does a defibrillator work?

> Delivers DC shock (AC causes myocardial damage and is arrhythmogenic).
> Uses 5000 V (this is much greater than that of the mains electricity and is produced using a step-up transformer).
> A capacitor is used to store charge. It consists of two conducting plates separated by an insulating material (dielectric). Capacitance is measured in farads (F). The amount of charge it can store depends on the size of the plates, their separating gap and the dielectric material. They have a low reactance to AC (i.e. passes AC) but a high resistance to DC (i.e. blocks DC).

$$\text{Charge (Q)} = \text{Capacitance (C)} \times \text{Voltage (V)}$$
$$\text{Energy stored (E)} = \tfrac{1}{2}\,CV^2$$

> An inductor is used to prolong the duration of current discharge (*see* Chapter 58, 'Electrical components'). It consists of coils of conducting material wound around a ferrous core (former). A magnetic flux is induced whenever a current flows through the coils causing back EMF and prolonging the charge. They have a high reactance to AC (i.e. block AC) but a low resistance to DC (i.e. pass DC).
> It produces a DC shock from 30 A, for 3 ms with 5000 V.
> The delivered (quoted) energy is less than stored charge due to some loss within the inductor.
> Thoracic impedance is in the region of 50–150 Ω. This is reduced after the first shock, by the use of conductive gel pads, front-to-back defibrillation and application of firm paddle pressure.
> External biphasic defibrillators deliver an energy of 150 J while monophasic ones deliver 360 J. Internal cardiac defibrillators (ICD) use 20–50 J.

How do cardioversion and defibrillation differ?

> During cardioversion, a synchronised DC shock must be administered in order to prevent 'R on T' phenomenon, which can trigger VF.
> During defibrillation of pulseless VT or VF, a non-synchronised shock can be administered.
> The energy delivered during cardioversion is often lower than for defibrillation e.g. 50 J for atrial fibrillation using a biphasic defibrillator, compared to 200 J for VF.

How can you calculate the energy that will be delivered during a shock?

This can be done using the equation $E = \frac{1}{2} CV^2$

> If C is 100 μF and V is 2000 V, then $E = \frac{1}{2} (0.0001)(2000^2) = 200$ J
> Energy stored will be 200 J.

In reality the energy delivered will be slightly less due to some loss within the system.

What are the safety considerations when using a defibrillator?

Use of a defibrillator necessarily means discharging a large amount of energy. If this is not done safely it can lead to:

> Burns.
> Ignition of flammable material and gases (fire and explosions).
> Interference with electrical components in contact with the patient such as ICDs and pacemakers.
> Precipitation of VF if shock intended to cardiovert is not synchronised correctly with patient's cardiac rhythm.
> Electrocution of staff and patient.

These risks can be minimised by:

> Allowing only trained personnel to deliver shocks.
> Ensuring all personnel are 'standing clear' when the shocks are delivered, i.e. not touching the patient and trolley/bed.
> Maintaining and checking defibrillator regularly.
> Having an audible alarm that signifies when defibrillator machine is 'charging' and 'ready to shock'.
> Having dry surroundings (patient and staff must not be in contact with fluid that can conduct the charge).
> Placing defibrillator pads on dry skin correctly to ensure maximal contact. If the pads are only partially in contact with the patient there will be a higher current density through the part that is in contact and this can lead to burns.
> Taking oxygen away/disconnecting it from the patient prior to delivery of shock.
> Having regular training and simulation sessions.

60. ELECTRICAL SAFETY

Questions on electrical safety do not have many places to go. However, that means that you do not have much room for manoeuvre if you do not know about it.

It is important to know about the different forms of electricity, the various circuit set-ups and the specific dangers of each in order to answer a question on safety measures with any confidence. Below are slightly wordier answers than you will have to give that should cover any selection of questions.

How is mains electricity supplied?

> Mains electricity is an alternating current (AC) supplied at 50 Hz and at 240 V.
> In AC, the flow of electric charge reverses direction periodically, producing a sine wave pattern.
> Electricity is delivered as AC to allow it to be transmitted over large distances (hundreds of miles) with very minimal loss of power. This is in sharp contrast to direct current (DC), which has a dramatic loss of power over just one mile.
> AC is generated at a voltage specific to the power plant generator. The voltage is then stepped up (using a transformer) to allow more efficient transfer of power over long distances before being stepped down (using a transformer) to 240 V for use.

What is the significance of the earth wire?

> UK mains electricity supply has three wires: live wire (brown), neutral wire (blue) and earth wire (green and yellow). Remember: 'Brown is Hot, Blue is Not, Green and Yellow earth the Lot'.
> The neutral wire is so called because it is connected to the earth at the mains transformer, so its electrical potential is 'neutral' with the earth.
> The live and neutral wires are relatively simple to understand but the earth wire often causes some confusion as on the one hand it is described as a safety measure but on the other hand it is imperative to protect the patient from exposure to earth. This is further complicated by the fact that the earth wire has different names like 'ground', which can mean different things in different circuits.
> The earth wire is a safety feature of electrical circuits designed to protect people from exposure to the full current of mains electricity in faulty appliances. It is a wire that literally returns to earth and completes a circuit with the generating power station and is connected to any exposed conducting parts of an electrical appliance.
> This means that if the live wire came into contact with a conducting part of the appliance, electricity would flow through the earth wire to earth. If the earth was not connected, someone touching the appliance would inadvertently act as a conduit for the electricity to flow and receive a severe shock. By having the earth there, the electricity flows preferentially down the earth wire (because earth is so large and therefore always offers the path of least resistance) rather than through the victim.

> Due to the deliberate application of tissue-damaging currents (diathermy) patients must be protected from contact with earth. If a patient was inadvertently connected to earth, they would provide an alternative route for the diathermy current to flow through, which could potentially cause severe burns at the point of contact between the patient and earth. Another safety reason to avoid patient contact with earth is to prevent the flow of leakage currents from faulty equipment through the patient.

What do the adverse effects of a current depend on?

> **Type of current:** AC is significantly more dangerous than DC. AC can cause tetanic muscular contractions ('can't let go' phenomenon) that peak at 50 Hz (frequency of mains electricity). This frequency is also particularly dangerous to the heart, making it prone to VF. With DC, there is a single muscle contraction, which typically throws the victim clear.
> **Magnitude of current** ($V = I \times R$)
> **Current density** (total current/area)
> **Current duration** (increased time means increased heat and hence increased tissue damage)
> **Tissues through which current flows** (cardiac muscle is prone to VF).

At what current amplitude would you feel tingling?

> 0–5 mA – tingling
> 5–10 mA – pain
> 10–50 mA – muscle spasm (15 mA 'can't let go' threshold)
> 50–100 mA – respiratory muscle spasm and VF
> 5 A – tonic contraction of the myocardium (this level of current is rarely seen except in defibrillation)

How can a pair of shoes keep you safe from current?

> This is all based on Ohm's law of $V = I \times R$.
> Resistance of skin is approximately 2000 Ω, body tissue is 500 Ω and shoes are 200 000 Ω.
> If a current was to enter skin, pass through body tissues and then exit through skin again, the total resistance it would encounter would be 4500 Ω (2000 + 500 + 2000).
> The magnitude of this current would therefore be:

I = V/R → 240/4500 → 53 mA (person at risk of arrhythmia)

> If current were to enter skin, pass through body tissues and then exit through shoes, the total resistance it would encounter would be 202 500 Ω (2000 + 500 + 200 000).
> The magnitude of this current would now be:

I = V/R → 240/202 500 → 1.2 mA (person would feel tingling sensation)

What is a macroshock?

Macroshocks are due to the passage of current from one part of the body to another (e.g. lightning or direct contact with a 'live' instrument whereby the body completes the circuit between the mains and earth). Current intensities required to cause harm are in the region of mA.

What is a microshock?

Microshocks are due to the passage of current directly to the myocardium (e.g. small leakage currents can pass through the heart via central lines, PA catheters and pacing wires). Current intensities required to cause harm are very small in the region of μA.

How is electrical equipment classified?

Electrical equipment is classified by its protection from mains electricity and by its allowable leakage current.

For mains protection it is classified as:

> **Class I** – earthed casing (all conducting surfaces are earthed)
> **Class II** – double insulated casing (no exposed conducting surface and so does not need to be earthed)
> **Class III** – battery-operated.

Electrical devices are designed to 'fail safe' and so if a single fault occurs no safety hazard should arise. Such conditions are called 'single fault conditions' (SFCs) e.g. the appearance of an external voltage on a part of equipment applied to the patient. When there is no fault the equipment is said to be in 'normal condition' (NC). Allowable leakage, of current is therefore defined under both sets of conditions.

For B and BF equipment, the patient leakage current is measured from all applied parts connected together and to earth.

B and BF: NC leakage current up to 0.1 mA
SFC Leakage current up to 0.5 mA

BF denotes a 'floating circuit' i.e. parts attached to the patient are isolated from the rest of the equipment e.g. ECG, ultrasound.

For CF equipment the current is measured from each applied part in turn and the leakage current must not be exceeded at any one applied part.

C   NC leakage current up to 0.01 mA
SFC leakage current up to 0.05 mA

What other measures are taken in theatre to prevent electrical injury?

> **Anti-static flooring** – this has high impedance to mains electricity but enough conductance to earth to prevent the build-up of static electricity.
> **Relative humidity of 50%** – inhibits the build-up of static electricity
> **Circuit breakers** – these consist of a transformer attached to a solenoid that will break a circuit or sound an alarm if a stray current above a set limit is detected flowing to earth.
> **Non-sparking switches and plugs**
> **Regular checks and maintenance of equipment**

61. DIATHERMY

What are the basic principles of diathermy?

> Diathermy devices are surgical instruments used to cut tissues and coagulate blood vessels.
> They use the heating effect of high frequency AC (0.5–1.0 MHz) passing through tissues of high impedance to burn or vaporise tissues in contact with the diathermy instrument.
> The heating effect of a current depends on the current density and duration.
> In diathermy the current density at the point where the instrument makes contact with the tissue is very high.
> In 'cutting' mode the current flows in an alternating sine wave pattern while in 'coagulation' mode the current flows in a pulsed sine wave pattern.
> Diathermy devices can either be monopolar or bipolar.
> In monopolar diathermy, current flows through a probe (active electrode) at a high current density and then returns via a diathermy plate (neutral plate) at low current density. The overall power that can be delivered is in the region of 100–400 W.
> In bipolar diathermy, the current is passed between two probes within a modified pair of forceps. One probe delivers the current and the second acts as the return circuit so tissues between the probes are exposed to the current and heated. This system helps keep the electrical field focal. The overall power this system can generate is approximately 40 W.

Why is the diathermy pad always checked at the end of surgery?

In bipolar diathermy the current makes a short journey across the tissue and is returned at a similar density, heating all the tissue between the electrodes. In monopolar diathermy the current exits at a point distant from the site of surgery, so it is important to ensure that the current density is low enough not to cause injury at this point. Hence the neutral plate has a large surface area and is applied over an area of good blood supply so that the current density is low and any heat generated can be dissipated by the blood flow. If the plate is not applied properly the reduced area or increased impedance can lead to more heat generation and burns, hence the reason the plate site is checked at the end of surgery.

What are the hazards of diathermy?

> **Burns**
> • Incorrect positioning of the neutral plate
> • Ignition of flammable skin preps
> • Inadvertent activation of diathermy probe (minimised by audible note when in use and use of a designated holder)

> **Electric shocks**
>   - Disconnection of the neutral plate may lead to current passing through an alternative route (e.g. ECG electrodes or exiting through a site where the patient may be in contact with a conducting surface). This can cause electrical shocks and burns to the patient.
> **Pacemaker interference**
>   - Ideally, diathermy should be avoided in patients with pacemakers and implantable cardioverter defibrillators (ICD) as electrical interference can cause these devices to malfunction.
>   - Pacemaker devices must be checked prior to surgery and alternative pacing techniques (external or transvenous) and cardiac arrest trolley should be available. ICDs should be disabled during surgery in which diathermy will be used.
>   - Surgical and theatre team must be informed.
>   - Bipolar is safer than monopolar diathermy.
>   - If monopolar diathermy is absolutely necessary, its use should be limited to short bursts of less than 5 seconds. The neutral plate must be well adhered and sited as far away from the pacemaker as possible.
>   - ECG monitoring is paramount.
> **Monitor interference**
>   - Diathermy interferes with monitoring including pulse oximetry, ECG and oesophageal Doppler.

What design features are incorporated within the diathermy system to minimise risk of electrical shock?

> **Use of an isolated patient circuit**
> **Use of an isolating capacitor:** Reactance of capacitors reduces with increasing current frequency; therefore, they have a higher impedance to low-frequency currents (i.e. they block conduction of AC and minimise the risk of macro- and microshocks) but a lower impedance to high-frequency diathermy currents (i.e. they allow conduction of these currents).

62. STATES OF MATTER, HEAT CAPACITY AND LATENT HEAT

Describe the difference between solids, liquids and gases.

Substances exist in the solid, liquid or gaseous state.

In the **solid** state a substance has a fixed shape, and the atoms or molecules of which it is composed are arranged in a regular pattern or lattice. In a molecular substance there are strong bonds between the atoms that make up the molecules and weaker bonds between the molecules themselves. The spacing between particles is at a minimum.

In a **liquid** state the substance has no fixed form; it takes up the shape of its container, but does not expand to fill it. Particles in a liquid constantly 'jiggle' about and the spacing between particles is slightly greater than that in the solid. Particles are free to move from one place to another in the liquid and there is no regular structure.

In a **gas** the particles are very far apart and move about in rapid random motion. A gas has no shape and completely fills any container. A gas which is below its critical temperature is called a **vapour**.

What causes a substance to change state?

At any time the state in which a substance exists depends on its composition and its temperature. In general, substances change state from solid to liquid to gas as the temperature rises. This is because the **temperature** is a measure of the average kinetic energy of the particles that make up the substance. It is the increase in energy possessed by the substance that causes the change of state.

As a solid is heated, it absorbs energy, which causes increased vibrations of the particles within it. Eventually, the kinetic energy of individual particles becomes so great as to overcome the inter-molecular forces holding the lattice together. The lattice breaks up in a process called **melting or fusion**.

Further heating results in more energy being given to the liquid particles until the last residual forces holding the particles in close contact are overcome and the particles separate widely, move randomly at high speeds and become a gas. This is **vaporisation**.

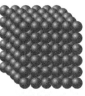

Solid   Liquid   Gas

Fig. 62.1　Molecular arrangement in solids, liquids and gases

What is 'heat capacity'?

The amount of energy given to a material to cause a 1 °C rise in temperature is called the heat capacity. There are two measures of heat capacity:

> The **Specific Heat Capacity** is defined as:
> • The amount of heat required to raise the temperature of 1 kg of a substance by 1 kelvin (or 1 °C)
> • The units are joule per kilogram per kelvin (J kg^{-1} K^{-1}).

> The **Molar Heat Capacity** is the amount of heat required to raise the temperature of 1 mole of the substance by 1 K (or 1 °C)
> • The units are joule per mole per kelvin (J mol^{-1} K^{-1}).

In general the more complex the chemical structure, the higher will be the heat capacity. This is because there are more ways for the molecule to vibrate in a complex molecule. Each mode of vibration can store kinetic energy. Therefore it takes more energy to heat it up by 1 degree.

Draw a graph to demonstrate the concept of latent heat and explain what happens when a solid is heated.

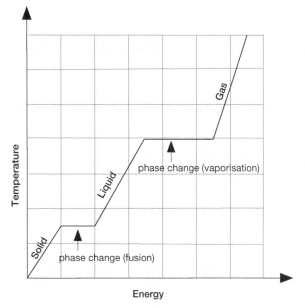

Fig. 62.2 Phase change with increasing energy

The diagram shows the rise in temperature as a solid is heated at a steady rate.

During the phase changes (fusion and vaporisation) the temperature remains constant even though heat is still being applied. This heat is used internally to overcome the attraction of the inter-molecular bonds. Work needs to be done to separate the particles against the forces of attraction. This heat is known as latent heat and the term comes from the Latin verb 'latere' – to lie hidden.

Latent heat refers to the amount of heat energy absorbed (or released) by a substance as it changes phase at a given temperature.

When going from solid to liquid (or vice versa) it is called the latent heat of fusion. When going from liquid to gas (or vice versa) it is called the latent heat of vaporisation.

> The **specific latent heat of fusion** of a substance is the heat required to convert 1 kg of solid at its melting point into liquid at the same temperature. The unit is joule per kilogram ($J\ kg^{-1}$).

> The **specific latent heat of vaporisation** of a substance is the heat required to convert 1 kg of liquid at its melting point into vapour at the same temperature. The unit is joule per kilogram ($J\ kg^{-1}$).

The specific latent heat of vaporisation is greater than that of fusion (seen on the graph) because more energy is required to overcome the intermolecular bonds here to liberate a gas.

A change of phase can be:

From solid to liquid	Fusion (Melting)
From liquid to vapour	Vaporisation
From vapour to liquid	Condensation
From liquid to solid	Freezing

The latent heat is given out to the surroundings when condensation or freezing occurs.

During melting or freezing the solid phase and the liquid phase are in equilibrium. During boiling the liquid and vapour phase are in equilibrium.

What clinical examples can you give where the concept of latent heat is important?

Use of ethyl chloride to provide local anaesthesia: vaporisation of the liquid phase of the agent from the surface of the skin causes cooling, rendering the sprayed area numb.

Use of volatile anaesthetic agents: vaporisation of the agent leads to cooling, which reduces the subsequent rate of vaporisation of the remaining agent and hence reduces the SVP. Vaporisers, therefore, have temperature compensation mechanisms (e.g. bimetallic strip that adjusts the splitting ratio) incorporated into their design to avoid fluctuations in the delivery of the volatile agent.

Use of nitrous oxide cylinder and liquid oxygen contained with a vacuum-insulated evaporator: vaporisation of these agents leads to cooling, which reduces the subsequent rate of vaporisation of the remaining agent and hence reduces the SVP.

Loss of latent heat from the patient through warming and humidification of inspired gases.

Loss of heat from the patient through evaporation.

A steam burn causes far more tissue damage than a burn from boiling water.

What is the triple point of water?

Please forgive the long-winded explanation, but we think this concept is explained poorly in other texts and merits a little more detail...

The states of a substance at different temperatures and pressures may be represented in a phase diagram. A typical phase diagram for a pure molecular substance is shown below.

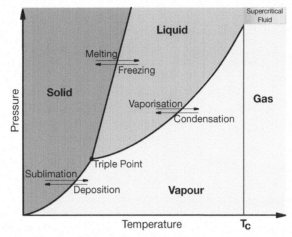

Fig. 62.3 Phase changes with pressure and temperature

The diagram shows the three states of matter – solid, liquid and gas.

You will see an area labelled 'supercritical fluid' on the diagram. A supercritical fluid is any substance at a temperature and pressure above its critical point, where distinct liquid and gas phases do not exist. A discussion of supercritical fluids is beyond the scope of this book and not necessary for the exam.

Above the triple point (see later), at a given pressure the substance progresses from solid to liquid to gas.

The boundaries between the three main areas of the phase diagram represent the conditions of temperature and pressure that two of the three phases are in equilibrium.

Thus along the solid/liquid boundary a solid is melting to a liquid. A small increase in pressure or a small decrease in temperature will cause the liquid to change back to solid and vice versa.

At the boundary itself there is a dynamic equilibrium where as many molecules of solid change to a liquid as molecules of liquid change to a solid.

Similarly along the liquid/vapour boundary, liquid is in equilibrium with vapour.

The solid/vapour boundary in the bottom left represents the equilibrium between solid and vapour. This is **sublimation**, where a solid changes to a vapour without going through the liquid phase. Solid carbon dioxide (dry ice) changes directly to the CO_2 vapour at normal atmospheric pressure.

The point at which the three boundaries meet is called the **triple point.** This is the point at which all three phases are in equilibrium.

For water, the triple point is 273.16 K (0.01 °C) at 611.73 Pa pressure (0.006 atm). The triple point of water is used as the upper fixed point in the definition of the kelvin scale of temperature.

How does boiling point change with pressure?

The boiling point of a substance increases with pressure. This is shown by the positive slope on the liquid/vapour boundary.

Similarly the melting point of most substances increases with pressure. Water is an exception; its melting point decreases with pressure. Its phase diagram actually has a negative slope for the solid/liquid boundary.

What is evaporation?

Particles of a liquid can move to the vapour state at any temperature. This is known as evaporation.

In a liquid the particles have kinetic energy and move about randomly in proximity to each other. Not all particles have the same amount of kinetic energy. Some will be moving slower and some will move faster. The distribution of energies of these particles is shown below:

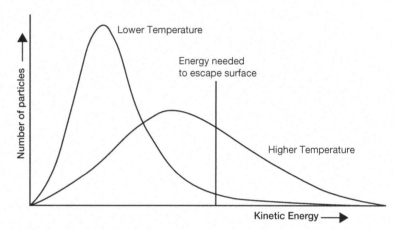

Fig. 62.4   Distribution of energy in particles in a liquid

A particle in the body of a liquid a will feel the attractive force of all the surrounding particles and will have no net force exerted upon it. However a particle near or at the surface of the liquid will have particles below it and to its side but none above it. Consequently, it will experience a net force inwards towards the body of the liquid; this is the origin of surface tension.

Evaporation occurs when a particle has sufficient energy to escape surface forces and move into the surroundings. At a low temperature only a small proportion of the particles will have sufficient energy to do this (*see* low-temperature energy curve above). At higher temperatures a greater proportion of particles have the required energy so evaporation is strongly dependent on temperature.

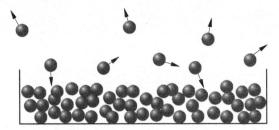

Fig. 62.5 Evaporation

Evaporation occurs only at the surface of a liquid. The particles that escape exert a pressure in the surroundings called the **vapour pressure**.

Explain the concept of saturated vapour pressure.

If a liquid is placed into a closed container, its molecules will evaporate and eventually a dynamic equilibrium will form between the number of particles escaping the liquid and the number rejoining in a given time. When this state is reached, the space above the liquid is saturated with vapour particles. These vapour particles will bounce off the surfaces of the container and of the liquid and in doing so exert a pressure.

This pressure is called the Saturated Vapour Pressure of the liquid (SVP).

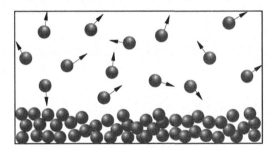

Fig. 62.6 Representation of saturated vapour pressure

Formally the SVP of a liquid is defined as:

• The pressure exerted by a vapour when in contact with and in equilibrium with its liquid phase within a closed system at a given temperature.

It is fairly obvious that heating the container, i.e. raising the ambient temperature, will raise the energy of the system and give more molecules sufficient energy to escape the surface of the liquid. Consequently, there will be a greater number of molecules bouncing against the sides of the container, resulting in a net increase in force, which is reflected in an increase in SVP. For a given substance in a closed system the SVP depends on temperature and nothing else (i.e. it is not affected by atmospheric pressure). The maximum SVP of an open system at sea level is 1 atmosphere.

How can the SVP of water at altitude cause hypoxia?

If atmospheric pressure at 5500 m above the sea level is $50 kP_a$ and saturated water vapour pressure is $6.3 kP_a$, the above question can be answered using the alveolar gas equation:

$P_{AMB}O_2 = F_{AMB}O_2 \times$ **Atmospheric pressure at altitude**
$= 0.21 \times 50 kP_a$
$= 10.5 kP_a$

$PiO_2 = F_{AMB}O_2 \times$ **(Atmospheric pressure at altitude − SVP of water)**
$= 0.21 \times (50 − 6.3)$
$= 9.17 kP_a$

$P_AO_2 = PiO_2 − P_ACO_2/RQ$
$= 9.17 − 5/0.8$
$= 2.92 kP_a$

What are the effects of SVP on a vaporiser?

As vapour is used up and removed from the vaporiser chamber it is replaced by further vaporisation of the volatile liquid.

The process of vaporisation requires energy (latent heat of vaporisation).

This energy requirement causes the temperature within the vaporiser to drop.

As SVP is dependent on temperature, this causes the SVP of the vapour to also drop.

In order to prevent this fluctuating SVP resulting in fluctuations in the delivery of volatile agent, vaporises have temperature-compensating mechanisms (e.g. bimetallic strip or heated vaporiser chambers).

What is boiling?

A liquid boils when the SVP equals the surrounding ambient pressure. This results in pockets, or bubbles, of vapour forming in the liquid and the liquid boils. These bubbles are less dense than the surrounding liquid and so rise to the surface, transferring energy to other liquid molecules they collide with on their way.

What are colligative properties?

Colligative properties are those properties of a solution that depend on the number of dissolved particles in a given mass of solvent and not on the identities and properties of those particles (i.e. they depend on the osmolality).

Freezing point – 1 mole of solute added to 1 kg of water will reduce its freezing point by 1.86 °C. This is why roads are gritted with salt during winter.

SVP – solute particles occupy space within the solvent, reducing the surface area available for vapourisation and hence reducing SVP.

Boiling point – this is the temperature at which liquid and vapour phases are in equilibrium but because solute particles occupy space within the solvent, the surface area available for solvent particles to enter the vapour phase is reduced. In order to re-establish equilibrium, the boiling point of the solution is achieved at a higher temperature.

Osmotic pressure – this is increased.

What is Raoult's law?

This law states that the depression of SVP of a solvent is proportional to the molar concentration of the solute present.

Why can't you 'have a nice cup of tea up Everest'?

Using the example of water in a saucepan at sea level, the ambient pressure is 1 atmosphere or $101.3 kP_a$. The water needs to be heated to 100 °C to attain sufficient energy to boil at this pressure. However, at the summit of Mount Everest, 8848 m above sea level, the ambient pressure is only 0.30 atmospheres or $30 kP_a$. It is easy to understand why up there, water only needs to be heated to around 80 °C to have sufficient energy to escape its liquid phase and boil and why you cannot have a 'nice hot cup of tea' at the top of Everest. In space, water cannot be boiled: it simply evaporates because the ambient pressure is very close to zero.

63. TEMPERATURE MEASUREMENT

What is heat?	Heat is a form of energy associated with the kinetic motion of molecules within a substance. Heat energy gets transferred from a hotter to a colder substance.
What is temperature?	Temperature refers to the thermal state of a substance. It is the degree of 'hotness' of a substance and reflects its potential for heat transfer.
What is the SI unit of temperature?	The standard international (SI) unit of temperature measurement is the kelvin (K). It is based on the triple point of water, which is the temperature (at a specific pressure) at which water exists in all three phases (273.16 K or 0.01 °C at a pressure of 611.73 Pa or 0.006 atm).

1 unit kelvin = 1/273.16 of the thermodynamic triple point of water.

A change in temperature of 1 K is equivalent to a change in temperature of 1 °C.

	From kelvin	To kelvin
Celcius	[°C] = [K] −273.15	[K] = [°C] +273.15

(All calculations must be performed using the kelvin scale and not celsius. The volume of a gas will double only if the absolute temperature doubles. So if the temperature increases from 283.15 K (10 °C) to 566.30 K (293.15 °C) the gas volume will double but this will not apply if the temperature doubles from 10 °C to 20 °C!)

What methods can be used to measure temperature?

Temperature measurement can be divided into non-electrical, electrical and infrared-based methods.

Non-electrical:
> **Liquid expansion thermometers** (e.g. mercury and alcohol thermometers):
  • **Principle:** Based on the volumetric expansion of a liquid with increasing temperature. Bulb containing the liquid is in communication with a narrow, linear, calibrated capillary tube. As the temperature increases the liquid expands and its volume increases causing it to rise up the capillary tube. An angled constriction prevents the liquid contracting back into the bulb until shaken. Alternatively, a small bobbin sitting above the liquid gets left at the maximum reading point until the device is shaken.
  • **Uses:** Mercury thermometers were previously used to measure body temperature (mercury freezes at about −39 °C and boils at about 250 °C) while alcohol thermometers are used to measure very low temperatures (alcohol freezes only at −114 °C and boils at 78 °C).
  • **Advantages:** Cheap and easy to use.
  • **Disadvantages:** Slow (2–3 min), glass thermometers can break causing injury and mercury is now classified as a hazardous substance.

> **Gas expansion thermometers** (e.g. Bourdon gauge dial thermometer):
  - **Principle:** Based on the volumetric expansion of a gas with temperature and the associated pressure changes that ensue due to this volume expansion. A bulb containing volatile liquid or saturated vapour is in communication with a hollow, elliptical, spiral tube. As the temperature rises, the volume in the bulb increases, and as the hollow tube tries to accommodate the expanded gas it changes shape from elliptical to circular in order to give it the largest possible cross-sectional area. This shape change causes the tube to uncoil, moving a pointer across a temperature scale.
  - **Uses:** Used outdoors in harsh environments.
  - **Advantages:** Cheap, robust and gives continuous measurements.
  - **Disadvantages:** Poor accuracy and requires recalibration.

> **Bimetallic strip dial thermometer:**
  - **Principle:** Coil consisting of two different metals with different expansion coefficients. As the temperature increases these metals expand by different amounts causing the coil to tighten and moving a pointer over the temperature scale.
  - **Uses:** Used outdoors in harsh environments.
  - **Advantages:** Cheap, robust and gives continuous measurements.
  - **Disadvantages:** Poor accuracy and requires recalibration.

> **Chemical thermometer:**
  - **Principle:** Strip of small cells containing a chemical mixture that melts over a range of temperatures to produce temperature-dependent colour changes. Newer reusable models use liquid crystal technology, where tiny colourless, solid crystals melt with increases in temperature and then realign themselves, causing a colour change.
  - **Uses:** Clinical body temperature measurement.
  - **Advantages:** Fast response time (<30 s), disposable and no risk of glass breakage.
  - **Disadvantages:** Not very accurate at temperature differences less than 0.5 °C.

Electrical:
> **Thermocouple:**
  - **Principle:** Consists of two different metals (e.g. copper and constantan, an alloy of copper and nickel) joined to form two separate junctions. One junction is kept at constant temperature and is known as the reference junction while the other junction acts as the temperature-measuring probe. When there is a temperature difference across these two junctions, a small voltage is produced. This voltage is proportional to the temperature difference across the junctions and is measured using a galvanometer. This phenomenon is known as the Seebeck effect.
  - **Advantages:** Rapid response time, accurate to within ±0.1 °C and small.
  - **Disadvantages:** Voltage produced is very small and needs signal amplification and the reference junction needs to be at a constant temperature (or requires compensation).

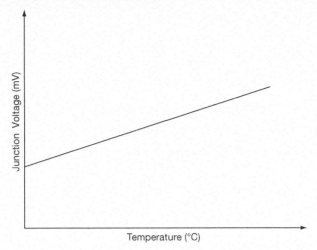

Fig. 63.1 Change in junction voltage (mV) vs. temperature (°C) for a thermocouple

> **Resistance thermometers** (e.g. platinum wire resistance thermometer):
  • **Principle:** Linear relationship between temperature and electrical resistance of a wire (e.g. platinum, copper or nickel) such that as temperature increases, the resistance within a platinum wire increases in a predictable manner.
  • **Advantages:** Extremely accurate to within ±0.0001 °C, with linear relationship between 0 and 100 °C.
  • **Disadvantages:** Slow response time, bulky and fragile.

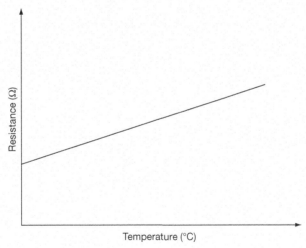

Fig. 63.2 Change in resistance (ohms) vs. temperature (°C) for a platinum resistance wire thermometer

> **Thermistor:**
  • **Principle:** Semiconductor composed of heavy metal oxide (e.g. nickel, iron or manganese) that displays a negative exponential relationship between electrical resistance and temperature.
  • **Uses:** Used clinically in PA catheters to measure core temperature.
  • **Advantages:** Rapid response time (<0.2 s), very small, accurate and cheap.
  • **Disadvantages:** Hysteresis, ageing, variability within a batch and non-linear relationship requires recalibration.

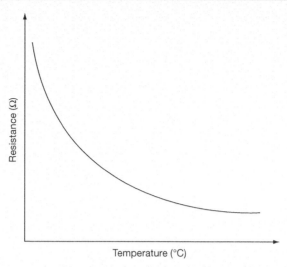

Fig. 63.3 Change in resistance (ohms) vs. temperature (°C) for a thermistor

Infrared:
> **Infrared tympanic membrane thermometers:**
  • **Principle:** All objects emit electromagnetic radiation, the wavelength
    of which is dependent on the temperature of that object. At body
    temperature, infrared radiation is the primary electromagnetic radiation
    given off by objects. Tympanic membrane thermometers receive
    infrared radiation from the tympanic membrane, which is close to the
    brain and therefore represents core body temperature. There are two
    main types of sensors that are used in these devices – the pyroelectric
    sensor and the thermopile sensor. The pyroelectric sensor contains
    crystals that alter their polarisation depending on the temperature. The
    thermopile sensor is made up of numerous thermocouples connected
    in series and allows continuous measurements to be made.
  • **Uses:** Clinical measurement of core body temperature.
  • **Advantages:** Non-invasive, accurate with a rapid response time (<5 s).

64. POLLUTION AND SCAVENGING

Delivery of anaesthesia may result in atmospheric contamination by anaesthetic gases such as nitrous oxide and volatile agents. In 1996 the Health and Safety Executive Agency placed constraints on the maximum allowable concentration of such substances within the theatre setting. In order to comply, scavenging of expired anaesthetic gases became mandatory.

What are the adverse effects of N_2O and volatile agents?

There are adverse effects to both the environment and staff (and patients).

Environment:
> Volatile agents and N_2O are both known to damage the ozone layer.
> N_2O is also a 'greenhouse' gas contributing towards global warming.
> N_2O sustains combustion and therefore in the presence of lasers or grease it can become a fire hazard.

Staff (adverse effects are primarily related to the use of N_2O):

> **Bone marrow toxicity and peripheral neuropathy:** N_2O inhibits the enzyme methionine synthase, which is involved in the synthesis of methionine (required for myelin formation) and tetrahydrofolate (required for DNA synthesis). It also oxidises the cobalt atom in vitamin B_{12} rendering it non-functional (vitamin B_{12} is a cofactor for methionine synthase). The result is megaloblastic changes in bone marrow, bone marrow suppression, megaloblastic anaemia, impaired spinal cord myelination (subacute combined degeneration of the cord) and peripheral neuropathy.
> **Teratogenicity:** Exact mechanism is unclear but is likely to be multi-factorial and involve impaired DNA synthesis, which can manifest as neural tube defects.
> **Spontaneous miscarriage:** There were reports suggesting an increased incidence of miscarriages in dental practice nurses working with N_2O. Although these reports got a lot of publicity there is still no good level of evidence to support this observation.
> **Substance abuse.**

What methods are available to reduce pollution in theatre?

> Air conditioning with rapid rate of air change (15 times per hour)
> Circle system
> Low gas flows
> Avoid using N_2O, use O_2 with air mix instead
> Scavenging systems
> Monitoring inspired and expired N_2O and volatile agent concentration and adjusting concentration to required clinical effect
> Monitoring theatre pollution levels

> Checking for leaks during daily anaesthetic machine check
> Capping breathing circuits when not in use (there is always a small leak)
> Vaporisers should be filled carefully to ensure no spillage
> Total intravenous anaesthesia technique
> Regional anaesthesia technique
> Rotate staff
> Regular servicing of anaesthetic machinery, gas supply, scavenging systems and ventilation
> Training and education of staff to be aware of potential hazards and how to minimise them

How can anaesthetic gases be scavenged?

Scavenging may be classified into active and passive systems.

Passive scavenging
> Requires no external power.
> Gas movement to the exterior is due to the pressure generated by the patient during expiration.
> This is an example of a ventile system (i.e. wind is used to entrain waste gases).

What are the problems with passive scavenging?

> Passive scavenging simply employs the use of wide-bore tubing to channel expired gases to the exterior and therefore it is not as effective as active methods.
> Excess positive or sub-atmospheric pressures may be caused by wind or air movement at the outlet.
> The outlets are above roof level to prevent re-entry of scavenged gas into the building; however, the weight of denser gases such as N_2O may exert a back-pressure into the patient's breathing system.

Active scavenging
> Utilises an external power source such as vacuum pumps to generate a negative pressure, which propels gases to the external atmosphere.

What are the components of an active scavenging system?

COLLECTING SYSTEM	[collection of expired gases from breathing system or ventilator]
↓	
TRANSFER SYSTEM	[wide-bore 30 mm tubing]
↓	
RECEIVING SYSTEM	[reservoir with visual flow indicator]
↓	
DISPOSAL SYSTEM	[air pump or fan generates a vacuum]
↓	
EXTERIOR	

> Gas from the expiratory valve of the breathing circuit or from the ventilator is collected and channelled via wide-bore, 30 mm diameter transfer tubing to the receiving system.
> The receiving system is usually an open-ended cylinder forming a reservoir for the collection of gases. The cylinder must be open-ended as a safety precaution, ensuring that the patient's airway cannot be subjected to excess positive or negative pressure.
> The receiving system also has a flow indicator. Scavenging flow rate is in the order of 80 L/min, which ensures removal of all expired gases.
> Gases in the reservoir are vented to the exterior atmosphere via a disposal system. The disposal system is either an air pump or a fan. It operates within a pressure of −0.5 to +5 cm H_2O.

What are the disadvantages of the active system?

> Excessive positive pressure may lead to barotrauma.
> Excessive negative pressure can deflate the reservoir bag of the breathing system and lead to rebreathing.

What is the recommended number of air changes per hour in theatre?

Despite scavenging, there will always be a quantity of gas that escapes into the theatre environment, and therefore the theatre needs adequate ventilation. Theatre ventilation should ensure 15 air changes per hour.

What is COSHH?

The Health and Safety Executive Agency is a government agency with the role of preventing death, injury and ill health in Britain's workplaces. COSHH – Control of Substances Hazardous to Health – sets safe maximum exposure limits to chemicals and other hazardous substances.

What are the maximum recommended anaesthetic pollutant levels?

These levels are based on an 8-hour TWA (time-weighted average).

Halothane	10 ppm
Enflurane	50 ppm
Isoflurane	50 ppm
Nitrous oxide	100 ppm
Sevoflurane	20 ppm (recommended limit by Abbot Laboratories)
Desflurane	No data provided

Are there any areas of the hospital in which long-term exposure limits may be difficult to achieve?

> It may be difficult to achieve acceptable pollution levels in post-anaesthesia care units – patients waking from anaesthesia with direct expiration into the environment of volatiles and possibly N_2O.
> Paediatric theatres – because of the use of non-closed breathing systems and high gas flows, e.g. Ayre's T-piece.

65. OXYGEN MEASUREMENT

There are multiple methods of measuring the concentration of oxygen in a gas mixture and it is essential to understand the principles behind each method.

How may the concentration of oxygen in a gas mixture be measured?

The different methods are:

> Clark polarographic electrode
> Galvanic fuel cell
> Paramagnetic O_2 analyser
> Mass spectrometer
> Photoacoustic spectroscope
> Raman spectroscope
> Chemical (e.g. Haldane apparatus).

Clark polarographic electrode:

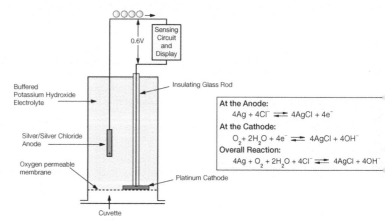

Fig. 65.1   The Clark electrode

> Silver/silver chloride (Ag/AgCl) anode and platinum (Pt) cathode are suspended within a potassium chloride (KCl) solution. Both are covered by an oxygen permeable membrane.
> Voltage of 0.6 V is applied across the electrodes to allow linearity between the current measured and the oxygen concentration in the sample.
> Flow of current is measured.
> Anode reaction: electrons (e^-) are generated by the reaction of Ag^+ with the Cl^- ions from the KCl solution.

> Cathode reaction: O_2 combines with e^- and water to generate hydroxyl (OH⁻) ions.

$$O_2 + 4e^- + 2H_2O \rightarrow 4OH^-$$

> The greater the amount of O_2 available, the greater the rate of electron uptake at the cathode and hence the greater the flow of current.
> Flow of current is therefore proportional to the O_2 tension at the cathode.
> Halothane may cause falsely high O_2 readings but this problem is overcome by the use of a halothane-impermeable membrane.
> The cathode has a lifespan of around 3 years because it becomes coated in protein. The membrane covering it helps to reduce protein deposition, but increases the response time of the electrode.
> The silver chloride anode will eventually be consumed.

Galvanic fuel cell:

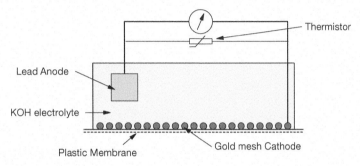

Fig. 65.2   The galvanic fuel cell

> Similar in principle to the Clark polarographic electrode.
> Gold (Au) mesh cathode and lead (Pb) anode are suspended within a potassium hydroxide (KOH) solution.
> Anode reaction: electrons are generated from the reaction between OH⁻ from KOH and the Pb anode.

$$Pb + 2OH^- \rightarrow PbO + H_2O + 2e^-$$

> Cathode reaction: O_2 combines with electrons and water to generate hydroxyl ions (i.e. same reaction for the Clark electrode).

$$O_2 + 4e^- + 2H_2O \rightarrow 4OH^-$$

> Unlike the Clark electrode, no battery is required as the fuel cell generates its own voltage.
> Response time of the system is slow at approximately 30 s and therefore not suitable for breath-to-breath measurements.
> Reagents are consumed limiting equipment lifespan to 6–12 months.
> The redox reaction at the cathode is temperature sensitive. Hence, temperature compensation is achieved using a thermistor.
> Gas mixtures containing N_2O may damage the fuel cell. N_2O reacts at the lead anode, generating N_2, which alters the pressure within the cell potentially causing damage.

Paramagnetic oxygen analyser:

> O_2 is a paramagnetic gas, which means that it is attracted towards a magnetic field because it has unpaired electrons in its outer shell. Most other gases (e.g. N_2) are diamagnetic and are repelled from magnetic fields.
> Analyser is composed of two nitrogen-filled glass spheres connected in a dumbell arrangement, suspended from a filament within a gas-tight chamber. A mirror is attached to the dumbell.
> Glass spheres are subjected to a non-uniform magnetic field.
> If O_2 is added to the chamber, it is attracted towards the magnetic field, causing rotation of the glass spheres.
> The degree of rotation of the glass spheres can be measured using a simple light beam deflection principle. A beam of light passing to the mirror gets deflected as the mirror rotates. This deflected beam is sensed by a photodetector, which is calibrated to match the degree of rotation of the system to the oxygen concentration within the chamber.
> Newer versions use the null deflection principle. Instead of the glass spheres rotating, a current is supplied to oppose the movement of the spheres. The amount of current required to keep the spheres in their resting position is calibrated to O_2 concentration.

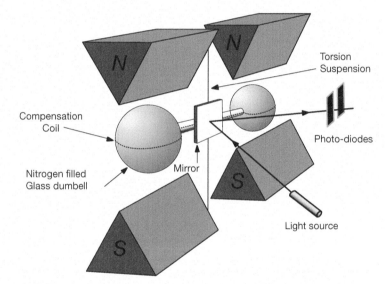

Fig. 65.3 The paramagnetic analyser

Mass spectrometer:

> Gas mixture is drawn into an ionising chamber where it is bombarded by electrons. As the electrons collide, they can knock off electrons from the gas molecules causing some of them to become charged.
> These charged particles are then accelerated through a strong magnetic field that deflects them to varying degrees depending on their mass and charge. The ion streams are measured at a detector plate, the number of plates determining how many gases can be measured.
> Compounds of identical molecular weight (MW) are distinguished by identifying their breakdown products, e.g. N_2O and CO_2 both have MW 44, so N_2O is identified from its smaller nitric oxide fragment (MW 30).
> A rapid response times of less than 0.1 s means mass spectrometry can be used for continuous gas analysis.
> It can measure a variety of gases within a mixture.
> Water vapour can interfere with the apparatus.
> It is a very bulky and an expensive piece of equipment.

Photoacoustic spectroscopy:

> Based on the photoacoustic effect, which was discovered by Alexander Graham Bell in his search for a means of wireless communication.
> Photoacoustic effect is the conversion between light and sound waves.
> Materials exposed to non-visible portions of the light spectrum (i.e. infrared and ultraviolet light) can produce acoustic waves.
> By measuring the sound at different wavelengths, a photoacoustic spectrum of a gas sample can be recorded and used to identify the components within that sample.
> This effect can be used to study solids, liquids and gases.

Raman spectroscopy:

> When light interacts with a gas molecule the rotational and vibrational energy of the molecule is altered during the interaction. The resulting transfer of energy to or from the light changes its wavelength by amounts characteristic of the molecule concerned. Monochromatic radiation is therefore changed during its passage through a gas sample chamber into a spectrum of wavelengths, which depends on the structure of the individual gas molecules. Thus the type of molecules present and their concentrations in the gas sample can be determined.
> Raman effect is the scattering of a photon in a gas. Raman scattering can occur with a change in vibrational, rotational or electronic energy of a molecule.
> Raman spectroscope is composed of a helium–neon laser as its radiation source, a gas sample cell and a set of eight detectors, each with a specific radiation wavelength filter.
> Filters are manufactured to measure O_2, N_2, CO_2, N_2O and certain volatile agents.

Haldane apparatus:

> This is utilised as an instrument for estimating the proportion of oxygen in expired gases.
> It consists of a burette containing a volume of gas.
> The gas is then exposed to a solution of pyrogallol (a powerful reducing agent able to absorb oxygen).
> The volume of the remaining gas is then measured.
> The reduction in gas volume indicates the quantity of oxygen absorbed by the pyrogallol.
> This system can also be used to measure CO_2, but here potassium hydroxide solution is used instead of pyrogallol.

66. pH MEASUREMENT

Define pH.

> pH stands for 'power of hydrogen'.
> It is a measure of the hydrogen ion activity in an aqueous solution.
> pH = negative log to the base 10 of the hydrogen ion concentration [H$^+$]:

$$pH = - \log_{10} [H^+]$$

There are a few rules of thumb worth remembering:

> Pure water is neutral and has a pH of 7.
> For each 1 unit change in pH there is a 10-fold change in [H$^+$].
> For each 0.3 change in pH there is a 50% change in [H$^+$].
> E.g.: pH 6 = [H$^+$] 1000 nmol/L or 10^{-6} mol/L
> pH 7 = [H$^+$] 100 nmol/L or 10^{-7} mol/L
> pH 7.4 = [H$^+$] 40 nmol/L or $10^{-7.4}$ mol/L
> pH 8 = [H$^+$] 10 nmol/L or 10^{-8} mol/L
> pH 9 = [H$^+$] 1 nmol/L or 10^{-9} mol/L.

How is [H$^+$] measured?

Arterial blood gas analysers measure [H$^+$] and PCO$_2$ using potentiometric electrodes (i.e. voltage-producing electrodes) and PO$_2$ via an amperometric technique (i.e. current-producing electrodes).

[H$^+$] is measured using a pH (glass) electrode, which is an ion-sensitive electrode whose operation depends upon the ion-sensitive glass at its tip.

It is an example of a potentiometric electrode in that a potential difference develops across the ion-sensitive glass, the potential difference being dependent upon the difference in [H$^+$] across the glass.

Draw a simple schematic pH electrode.

> Reference electrode: mercury/mercury chloride electrode within a potassium chloride solution. This solution is saturated and acts as a salt bridge to complete the circuit between the sample and the electrode. The KCl solution is prevented from diffusing into the sample by a porous membrane that is permeable to only H$^+$ ions.
> pH electrode: silver/silver chloride electrode within a buffer solution of hydrochloric acid. The tip of the electrode is composed of pH-sensitive glass.
> The temperature of the system is maintained at 37 °C because dissociation of acids and bases increases with increasing temperature.

> [H⁺] is held constant around the pH electrodes by the buffer solution and so any potential difference across this electrode is due to [H⁺] within the blood sample.
> Potential difference between the two electrodes is measured and converted to a direct reading of pH or [H⁺].
> Potential output is linear (60 mV per unit pH).

pH Electrode

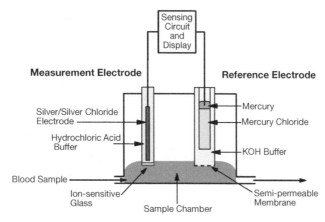

Fig. 66.1 The pH electrode

How is the pH electrode calibrated?

The pH scale is not an absolute scale; it is relative to a set of standard solutions whose pH has been established by international agreement. The system is calibrated using two of these standard buffer solutions of known pH.

What are the sources of error in this measuring system?

The following conditions may result in erroneous [H⁺] results:

> Calibration errors
> Drift of the measuring system
> Membrane damage resulting in electrode contamination
> Temperature – hypothermia increases CO_2 solubility resulting in reduced $PaCO_2$ and increased pH
> Sampling errors
> Effect of over-heparinisation – acidic heparin lowers pH.

Delays in analysis of arterial blood gas – cellular metabolism continues:

> PCO_2 rises about 0.009 kP$_a$ per minute
> pH falls approximately 0.0006 units per minute
> PO_2 falls approximately 0.13–0.39 kP$_a$ per minute.

What other method can be used to measure pH?

A pH indicator is a substance that will change colour at a particular pH value (e.g. litmus paper turns red in acidic and blue in alkaline conditions).

67. CARBON DIOXIDE MEASUREMENT

How is CO₂ measured in solution? Carbon dioxide (CO_2) is routinely measured in anaesthetic practice:

> Arterial blood gas analysis (partial pressure of CO_2 in the blood)
> Capnography (percentage CO_2 in expired gas).

CO₂ is measured in solution using the Severinghaus or CO_2 electrode.

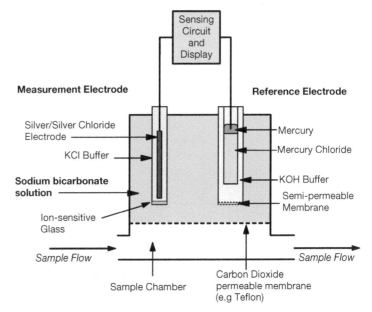

Fig. 67.1 The Severinghaus CO_2 electrode

> Measurement of PCO_2 is based upon [H⁺] measurement.

$$CO_2 + H_2O \leftrightarrow H_2CO_3 \leftrightarrow H^+ + HCO_3^-$$

> The CO_2 electrode is a modified pH electrode in contact with sodium bicarbonate solution. It is kept separate from the blood sample to be analysed by a semi-permeable membrane.
> CO_2 is able to diffuse across this membrane and react with H_2O to generate H⁺ ions. The resulting change in [H⁺] is measured by the glass electrode (potentiometric electrode).
> Response time of the system is in the order of 2–3 min.
> It requires calibration prior to use with gas of known CO_2 concentration.
> The temperature of the system must be maintained at 37 °C.

How is CO_2 measured in a gas mixture?

Capnography has become an integral part of monitoring in anaesthesia. Monitors can use infrared spectrography, mass spectrography, Raman spectrography, photoacoustic analysers (*see* Chapter 65, 'Oxygen measurement' for details of these techniques) or colorimetric devices to measure carbon dioxide in the respiratory gases and then give a numerical reading (capnometry) and a waveform (capnography). We will look at the most commonly used monitor, the infrared analyser.

Infrared analyser
> Diatomic gas molecules (i.e. containing two or more different atoms) absorb infrared radiation.
> Each diatomic gas absorbs radiation of a particular wavelength.
> By measuring the proportion of infrared radiation absorbed by a gas mixture, the partial pressure of a diatomic gas can be inferred.
> An infrared beam passes through a filter to obtain the required frequency of light absorbed by the gas of interest.
> The infrared beam splits and passes through reference and sample gas chambers.
> Sample and reference chamber windows are made of crystal (silver bromide or sapphire) as glass absorbs infrared.
> CO_2 absorbs infrared radiation and emergent beams are compared by photoelectric cells (the detector).
> The analyser is calibrated using air (assumed zero CO_2) and a known concentration of CO_2 (gas cylinder) or electronically (step input voltage).
> Analysis is affected by the barometric and extraction pressure in system – a change in atmospheric pressure directly influences the reading of capnographs since CO_2 concentration is measured as partial pressure.
> A water vapour trap is required (water has high infrared absorbance).
> Hygroscopic tubing is needed.

If you were allowed only one anaesthetic monitoring device, what would you chose?

Most anaesthetists would probably request capnography because of the amount of information that can be gained from capnogram analysis:

> Confirmation of endotracheal intubation
> Detection of rebreathing (inadequate fresh gas flow)
> Detection of obstructive expiratory airflow
> Detection of inter-breathing in a ventilated patient
> Sudden fall in end-tidal CO_2 may indicate low systemic blood pressure, circulatory arrest or pulmonary embolism
> End-tidal CO_2 provides an estimation of arterial $PaCO_2$
> Detection of malignant hyperpyrexia

Which parameters are measured directly by an arterial blood gas analyser?

Directly measured:

> PaO_2
> $PaCO_2$
> pH

Derived:

> HCO_3^-
> base excess
> O_2 saturations

68. BLOOD PRESSURE MEASUREMENT

This is a common question both in the primary and final FRCA exam. Good basic understanding of the principles underlying BP measurement is essential.

How can you measure blood pressure?

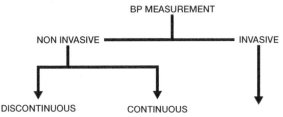

BP MEASUREMENT

NON INVASIVE ——————— INVASIVE

DISCONTINUOUS
- Manual occlusive cuff method (Riva-Rocci or Korotkoff)
- Von Recklinghausen oscillonometer
- Automated occlusive cuff method

CONTINUOUS
- Penaz technique
- Doppler ultrasound

- Arterial line with piezoresistive strain gauge (*see* Chapter 69, 'Arterial pressure waveform')

Describe the manual occlusive cuff method.

This uses a cuff most commonly placed around the upper limb. The cuff must cover two-thirds of the length of the limb (or it must be 20% greater that the diameter of the limb). The width of a standard adult cuff is 14 cm and the cuff length should be twice the width. If the cuff is too small it will over-read and if too large it will under-read.

> **Riva-Rocci method:** Blood pressure was measured by palpation of the brachial or radial artery as the cuff was inflated. The loss of the pulse represented systolic blood pressure. Riva-Rocci (an Italian physician) was credited with developing the first conventional sphygmomanometer.

> **Korotkoff method:** Blood pressure was measured by auscultation over the brachial artery. In 1905, Korotkoff (a Russian army surgeon) described a series of noises that could be heard over the brachial artery as the cuff deflated:
> - **Phase I:** Tapping sound appears (systolic blood pressure)
> - **Phase II:** Sounds muffle or disappear (auscultatory gap)
> - **Phase III:** Sounds reappear with a tapping quality
> - **Phase IV:** Sounds muffle again (diastolic blood pressure in the UK)
> - **Phase V:** Sounds disappear (diastolic blood pressure in the USA). In a hyperdynamic circulation, the sounds may never disappear and this is why we use phase IV to denote diastolic pressure.

What are the advantages and disadvantages of using this method?

Advantages:
> Simple
> No electricity required
> Doctor–patient contact

Disadvantages:
> Operator dependent
> Correct cuff size required
> Artefacts with arrhythmias and movement
> Tourniquet effect can cause nerve damage
> Underestimates hypertension and overestimates hypotension

How does a von Recklinghausen's oscillotonometer work?

The old-fashioned versions of these machines work using two cuffs. The first is an occluding cuff, which sits proximally, and the second a sensing cuff against which the blood pulses once the occluding cuff has been deflated sufficiently to allow blood to flow under it. Each cuff is attached to two bellows and these bellows are attached to a single needle. A lever enables the operator to select which bellow's pressure is displayed by the needle (i.e. it can either make the needle 'sensing' or 'reading' depending on which position it is in).

> At systolic blood pressure – there is a sudden increase in needle oscillations.
> At mean arterial pressure – there is maximal amplitude in needle oscillations.
> At diastolic blood pressure – there is a sudden decrease in needle oscillations.

How does a 'DINAMAP' work?

DINAMAP® is the trade name for one of the original automated occlusive BP cuff measuring devices. It is based on the principle of an oscillotonometer, but now the two cuffs have been merged into a single cuff, which performs both occluding and sensing functions. There is also a pneumatic pump, bleed valve, transducer, processor and display monitor.

> As the cuff deflates, the transducer detects the flow of blood under the cuff.
> The processor, with a built-in algorithm, then relates the rate of change of pressure transients to systolic, diastolic and mean blood pressures.
> These readings are then displayed on the monitor.

Describe the Penaz technique (the 'Finapres').

Penaz principle states that 'the force exerted on a body can be determined by measuring an opposing force that prevents physical disruption'. It consists of an infrared plethysmograph within a pneumatic cuff.

> The Finapres cuff is wrapped around the distal phalanx of a finger (over a digital artery). It shines an infrared light through the finger, which is detected on the opposite side. The amount of light absorbed is directly proportional to the volume of the finger (this volume changes during systole and diastole).
> A pneumatic pump is controlled by the infrared signal. It continuously adjusts the cuff pressure in order to maintain a constant infrared signal (it aims to keep the volume of the finger constant, which represents the mean arterial pressure).
> The pressure inside the cuff required to achieve this is measured and gives a continuous arterial BP reading.

What are the advantages and disadvantages of this method?

Advantages:
> Continuous reading
> Accurate

Disadvantages:
> Downward drift due to tissue fluid relocation
> Painful after 20–30 min
> Ischaemia of digit

How can Doppler ultrasound be used to measure BP?

This is based on the principle of the Doppler shift.
> Transducer crystals within a probe transmit and receive ultrasound waves.
> Probe positioned over artery with a coupling medium (e.g. gel).
> As the arterial wall moves during systole and diastole there is a Doppler shift in frequency of the ultrasound waves (*see* Chapter 80, 'Ultrasound and Doppler').

69. ARTERIAL PRESSURE WAVEFORM

What are the indications for direct arterial blood pressure measurement?

> When non-invasive BP measurements are inaccurate – in obese patients, arrhythmias and during ambulance transfers.
> When extreme changes in blood pressure are expected – massive haemorrhage, cardiovascular instability and induced hypotension.
> When frequent arterial blood samples are required.
> When using pulse-contour cardiac output monitoring (e.g. LiDCO).

What are the components of an arterial line used to measure blood pressure?

> **Arterial cannula**: short, stiff and 20 G size in adults.
> **Tubing:** usually less than 120 cm, filled with 0.9% saline, connects cannula to transducer, must be free of kinks, clots and air bubbles.
> **Three-way tap and flushing device.**
> **Pressurised fluid bag:** usually 0.9% saline, pressurised to 300 mmHg, with a drip rate of 4 mL/h to prevent clot formation within the cannula.
> **Diaphragm:** very thin membrane acts as an interface between the transducer and the fluid column.
> **Piezoresistive strain gauge transducer connected to a Wheatstone bridge circuit** (a null-deflection system consisting of a galvanometer, two constant resistors, one variable resistor and a strain gauge)**:** must be zeroed to atmospheric pressure and kept at the level of the right atrium.
> **Microprocessor, amplifier and display unit**

What factors determine the shape of the arterial waveform?

> Volume of blood ejected
> Speed at which this blood is ejected during each beat
> Ability of the vascular tree to distend and accommodate this ejected blood (i.e. compliance of arterial tree)
> Rate at which this ejected blood is able to flow from central arterial component into the peripheral tissues (i.e. systemic vascular resistance)

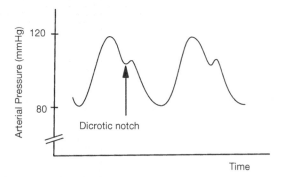

Fig. 69.1 Arterial pressure waveform

What information can be derived from a direct arterial pressure wave?

> Systolic blood pressure: this is primarily influenced by stroke volume and compliance. This explains why elderly patients have a higher systolic pressure due to a reduced vascular compliance secondary to atherosclerosis while neonates have a lower systolic pressure because of a very compliant arterial tree.
> Diastolic blood pressure: this is primarily influenced by arterial recoil. This explains why elderly patients have a lower diastolic pressure as their stiff arteries are not able to recoil effectively while neonates have a higher diastolic pressure due to their good arterial elastic recoil.
> Pulse pressure
> Mean arterial pressure
> Heart rate
> Rhythm
> Dicrotic notch: this represents the nadir point that occurs immediately after the aortic valve closes and is usually seen one-third of the way down the descending limb of the pressure wave (i.e. when pressure in aorta is greater than the pressure in left ventricle). The position of this notch reflects peripheral vascular resistance. In presence of vasodilatation (e.g. sepsis or epidural), there is a downward shift of the dicrotic notch. Characteristic features of vasodilatation of the arterial wave form include a low systolic pressure, low diastolic pressure, wide pulse pressure and delayed dicrotic notch.
> Left ventricular contractility: this can be estimated from the gradient of the upstroke of the arterial waveform.
> Compliance of the arterial tree: this can be estimated from the gradient of the downstroke of the arterial waveform.
> Stroke volume: this can be estimated from the area under the systolic portion of the arterial waveform (i.e. from the start of the upstroke to the dicrotic notch).
> Heart–lung interactions and fluid responsiveness: the changes in arterial pressure waveforms in response to changes in intra-thoracic pressures during mechanical ventilation (i.e. 'swing') can be used to determine fluid responsiveness.
> Pulse contour analysis can be used to determine stroke volume and cardiac output (for more details, *see* Chapter 70, 'Cardiac output monitoring').

In what ways can a direct arterial pressure transducer system give you false information?

> **Calibration error:** one-point calibration is suitable for highly accurate devices to remove the offset error. Two-point calibration is required for less accurate devices but with an assumed linear response, in order to remove offset and gain errors. Three-point calibration is used for devices that are not very accurate or that have a very non-linear response. Arterial lines undergo a one-point calibration by zeroing the transducer to atmospheric pressure. However, despite calibration, drift of zero and gain can occur over time.
> **Transducer height:** this must be at the level of the patient's right atrium (an error reading equivalent to 7.5 mmHg occurs for each 10 cm discrepancy in height).
> **Natural frequency and resonance:** every system has a tendency to oscillate. When a system is given a small oscillation (an external push), it will start to swing and the frequency at which it swings is the natural frequency (also called resonant frequency) of that system. Natural frequency is directly related to resonance. It is important for the natural frequency of the arterial transducer to be significantly different from the frequency of the arterial pressure wave or else it could amplify the signal (natural frequency should be at least 10 times fundamental frequency).

Natural frequency is:
- Directly related to catheter diameter
- Inversely related to square root of the system compliance
- Inversely related to the square root of the length of tubing
- Inversely related to square root of the density of the fluid in the tubing.

> **Frequency response:** arterial pressure waveform is a complex sine wave. Fourier analysis allows this complex waveform to be broken down into a series of simple sine waves of different amplitudes and frequencies. The fundamental frequency (or first harmonic) is equal to the heart rate (HR of 60 bpm = 1 Hz, HR of 120 bpm = 2 Hz and so on). The first 10 harmonics of the fundamental frequency contribute to the waveform, and therefore, in order to display the arterial waveform correctly, the transducer should have a frequency response range (i.e. bandwidth) of 0.5–40 Hz.

> **Damping:** this is the tendency of an object to resist oscillating (*see* Chapter 52, 'Principles of measurement', for more details). Over-damping underestimates SBP, overestimates DBP but MAP remains the same (e.g. blood clot, air bubble or excessive tubing compliance). Under-damping overestimates SBP, underestimates DBP but MAP remains the same (e.g. tubing too long and non-compliant). In order to minimise these errors, the monitoring system should apply an optimal damping value of 0.64.

What are some of the complications associated with arterial lines?

> Cannula disconnection leading to blood loss
> Arterial thrombosis
> Ischaemia distal to the cannula (this is rare but can occur so collateral circulation should be checked, e.g. Allen's test)
> Infection
> Inadvertent drug administration: this can cause distal vascular occlusion and ischaemia. A-lines should be clearly labelled and colour-coded.

70. CARDIAC OUTPUT MONITORING

Cardiac output (CO) is defined as the volume of blood ejected from the left ventricle per minute. It is determined by a number of interplaying factors including heart rate, rhythm, preload, contractility and afterload. Circulation (both in terms of pressure and flow) is essential to organ perfusion and O_2 delivery. However, it varies significantly under different physiological extremes and disease states.

Cardiac output monitoring measures various parameters associated with the central circulation and is currently the Holy Grail of haemodynamic assessment. Over the last decade there has been a rapid expansion in the use of CO monitoring devices within critical care and theatre settings to aid optimisation of haemodynamic variables and O_2 delivery and to facilitate goal-directed therapy CO monitoring is also essential to many enhanced recovery programmes.

The ideal method of measuring CO would be non-invasive, accurate, continuous, safe, easy to use and operator independent. It would provide rapid data acquisition and be cost-effective. Unfortunately, none of the currently available CO monitoring devices possesses all these properties.

Conventional thermodilution techniques using a pulmonary artery floatation catheter (PAFC) remain the clinical gold standard for accuracy in CO monitoring. However, newer, less invasive monitoring devices that provide continuous CO data are establishing a role in haemodynamic management.

What methods are available to measure cardiac output?

> Fick's principle
> Thermal/indicator dilution techniques
> Doppler ultrasound
> Electrical bioimpedance
> Arterial pulse pressure contour analysis

What is the Fick's principle?

Fick (a nineteenth-century German physiologist, credited for Fick's law of diffusion and the invention of the contact lens) identified that the uptake or release of a substance (M) by an organ is the product of the blood flow (Q) through that organ and the arteriovenous concentration difference (A-V) of the substance in question.

$$M = Q \times (A\text{-}V)$$

In essence, the Fick's principle allows the blood flow to an organ (or the body) to be calculated using a suitable marker substance (e.g. dye, temperature or O_2).

How can you calculate CO using the Fick's principle?

> The Fick method of calculating CO uses the Fick's principle to measure the CO of the pulmonary circulation.
> The A-V oxygen content difference across the lungs is measured via arterial and venous blood gases (i.e. a mixed venous sample from the pulmonary artery) and the rate of oxygen uptake is measured via spirometry.

$$\dot{V}O_2 = CO \times (CaO_2 - C\bar{v}O_2)$$

and therefore

$$CO = \dot{V}O_2/(CaO_2 - C\bar{v}O_2)$$

Where:

$\dot{V}O_2$ = oxygen uptake
CaO_2 = arterial oxygen content
$C\bar{v}O_2$ = mixed venous oxygen content
CO = cardiac output

> In the absence of intra-pulmonary or intra-cardiac shunts, the pulmonary blood flow is equal to systemic blood flow and thus cardiac output.

What do you understand by the term 'assumed Fick determination'?

The Fick's method is extremely accurate, but in reality it is very time-consuming and cumbersome to obtain the required measurements. Therefore, the assumed value for O_2 consumption (250 mL/min or 125 mL/min/m^2) is sometimes used to calculate the CO. This is called an assumed Fick determination.

How is the dye or indicator dilution technique used to measure CO?

> A known quantity of dye (e.g. indocyanine green) or indicator substance (e.g. lithium) is injected into a central vein and then measured distally from a peripheral arterial blood sample.
> A graph of concentration over time is then plotted.
> Due to recirculation of the substance, a second peak known as a 'recirculation hump' is seen on the concentration–time curves and this limits the total number of measurements that can be taken.
> The graph is therefore plotted semi-logarithmically in order to minimise the effect of this recirculation.
> The CO is inversely related to the area under the curve (AUC).
> Computer algorithms use the modified Stewart–Hamilton equation to calculate CO.

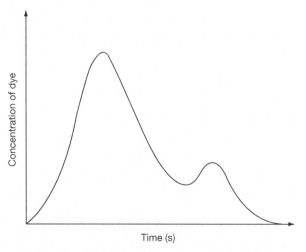

Fig. 70.1 Concentration of dye over time

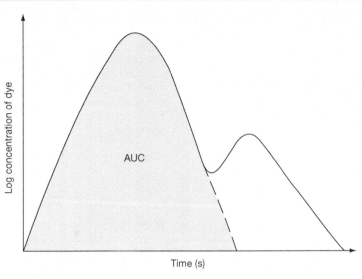

Fig. 70.2 Log concentration of dye over time

What is a pulmonary artery flotation catheter (PAFC)?

> A PAFC is a device that can be used to measure cardiac filling pressures, pulmonary artery occlusion pressure, central venous oxygen saturations and core temperature.
> Cardiac output data may be acquired through thermodilution methods using the PAFC.
> Global use of the PAFC is falling as a result of newer, relatively less invasive methods of CO monitoring becoming available. Nevertheless, the PAFC is an extremely accurate method of CO monitoring and newer monitoring devices are routinely validated against the PAFC thermodilution technique.

Describe the key features of the PAFC.

> 110 cm long, balloon-tipped, flow-directed catheter.
> Inserted via a 5 FG introducer sheath
> Distal lumen should be positioned in the pulmonary artery (PA) to allow measurement of PA pressure and allow sampling of mixed venous blood.
> Proximal lumen is 30 cm from distal tip and should be positioned in the right atrium.
> Balloon at the tip is inflated with up to 1.5 mL of air (necessary to allow the catheter to advance with blood flow and to enable measurement of pulmonary capillary wedge pressure).
> Cardiac output is measured using cold thermodilution or pulsed heating bursts (latter available only in newer catheters).
> Pulmonary capillary wedge pressure (PCWP) provides an indication of left atrial filling pressure and thereby left ventricular end-diastolic pressure (LVEDP), which is used as a surrogate for left ventricular end-diastolic volume (LVEDV) that represents preload.

How is cardiac output measured using a PAFC?

> A thermodilution technique is used (which is an advance on the dye dilution technique) where heated or cooled fluid is now used to replace the dye. This eliminates the problems of recirculation, allowing infinite measurements to be made.
> 10 mL ice-cold 0.9% saline (or 5% dextrose) is injected via the proximal port of the PAFC into the right atrium, thereby reducing the blood temperature.
> The blood temperature is then measured by a distal thermistor on the PAFC and a thermodilution curve (temperature change against time) is generated.

> Cardiac output is inversely related to the AUC and computer programmes calculate it using the **Stewart–Hamilton equation**:

$$Q = \frac{V(T_B - T_1)K_1K_2}{T_B(t)dt}$$

Where:

Q   cardiac output
V   volume of injectate
T_B temperature of blood
T_1 injectate temperature
K_1K_2 computer constants
$T_B(t)dt$ change in blood temperature over time

> Modern PAFCs are able to provide continuous CO data. They contain an electric heating coil that is positioned in the right atrium and which heats up the blood in a semi-random manner. The pulsed heating bursts are detected by the thermistor, and via the same Stewart–Hamilton method CO is calculated.

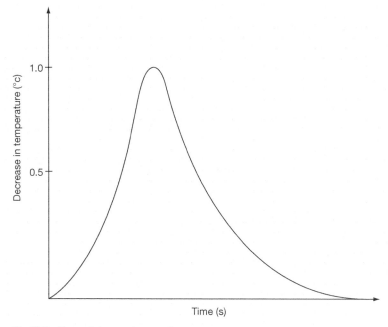

Fig. 70.3   Change in temperature over time

Draw a pressure trace to illustrate the PAFC passage to the pulmonary artery.

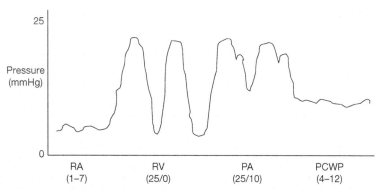

Fig. 70.4   PAFC passage through the heart

In what circumstances does PCWP overestimate LVEDP?

Any condition creating an interfering pressure gradient that does not represent function of the left ventricle:
> Mitral stenosis
> Positive end expiratory pressure (PEEP)
> Pulmonary hypertension

In what circumstances does PCWP underestimate LVEDP?

Any condition causing increased pressure within the left ventricle, which the catheter tip cannot detect:
> Poorly compliant left ventricle
> LVEDP >25 mmHg

How is a PCWP of 25 mmHg interpreted?

> The most common interpretation of an elevated PCWP in the assumed setting of normal juxtacardiac pressure and normal ventricular compliance would be that of hypervolaemia with an increased LVEDV causing an elevated PCWP.
> If juxtacardiac pressure is increased, as in cardiac tamponade or constrictive pericarditis, the same elevated PCWP may be associated with normal or reduced LVEDV.
> Another scenario is possible if ventricular compliance is reduced (e.g. diastolic dysfunction arising from myocardial ischaemia), in which case again LVEDV may be normal or reduced despite elevated PCWP.
> These problems delineate the basis of arguments that are now made against the use of PCWP as a marker of fluid responsiveness.

What other methods of cardiac output measurement do you know of?

Examiners will expect an understanding of the principles behind cardiac output monitoring and may wish to explore the advantages and disadvantages of some of the commoner technologies available.

Non-invasive techniques:
> **Transcutaneous Doppler** (e.g. ultrasound cardiac output monitor – USCOM)
  • Based on the Doppler effect.
  • Transcutaneous probe is placed on the supra-sternal notch of the patient.
  • Measures blood flow in the pulmonary artery and across the semi-lunar valves.
  • Device plots velocity of trans-valvular and trans-pulmonary blood flow over time.
  • Programmed algorithms within the device then calculate the CO.
  • User-dependent and requires training.

> **Transthoracic electrical bioimpedance**
  • Based on the principle that during ejection of blood from the heart in systole there is an associated change in electrical impedance of the thoracic cavity due to the increased blood volume, the rate of change of this impedance is a reflection of CO.
  • Four dual electrodes or sensors are placed on the neck and thorax and a low current is passed between them.
  • Current seeks the path of least resistance, which in this case is the blood-filled aorta.
  • Blood volume and velocity within the aorta changes from beat to beat and this equates to changes in thoracic impedance.
  • Device measures the corresponding changes in impedance and relates these to CO.
  • Quick to set up and easy to use.
  • Useful in estimating trends in CO but not for absolute measurements.
  • Studies suggest the method is accurate in healthy volunteers, but its reliability decreases in critically ill patients.
  • Technique has not gained wide clinical acceptance.

> **Non-invasive cardiac output monitor (NICO)**
- Applies the Fick's principle to CO_2.
- Changes in CO_2 concentration after intermittent periods of partial rebreathing through a special rebreathing loop are measured.
- Sensors are placed to measure CO_2, air flow and airway pressures.
- $\dot{V}CO_2$ is calculated from minute ventilation including its CO_2 content while $PaCO_2$ is estimated from end tidal CO_2 measurements.
- System relies solely on airway gas measurement.
- Calculates effective lung perfusion (i.e. that part of the pulmonary capillary blood flow that has passed through ventilated parts of the lung).
- Effects of unrecognised ventilation–perfusion inequality in patients may explain why the results with this method show a lack of agreement with thermodilution techniques.

Invasive techniques:
> **Transoesophageal Doppler**
- Based on the Doppler effect.
- Velocity of blood flow in the descending thoracic aorta is measured using a flexible ultrasound probe placed in the mid-oesophagus. The frequency change (Doppler shift) measured correlates directly with the speed of blood travelling in the aorta.
- The integral of the blood velocity–time waveform (area under the curve) then represents stroke distance.
- This waveform is displayed on the monitor and, in addition to the associated sound of the waveform, can help in positioning the probe.
- The product of the cross-sectional area of the aorta and the stroke distance gives the stroke volume (nomograms are used to calculate diameter of the descending aorta, based on height, age and weight).
- Provides indicator of preload (flow time corrected to 60 beats per min) and contractility (peak velocity and mean acceleration).
- Systemic vascular resistance is calculated.
- Rapid data acquisition.
- Only measures blood flow in the descending aorta and hence flow to head, neck and upper limbs is excluded.
- Not tolerated by awake patients.
- Suffers interference from surgical diathermy.
- Operator dependent and requires skill to align probe and obtain good signal.
- Contraindicated in those with oesophageal varices.
- Risk of oesophageal perforation.

> **Dye and temperature dilution techniques** (covered previously)

> **Arterial pulse contour analysis** (e.g. PiCCO and LiDCO)
- The size of the pulsatile component of the arterial waveform (the pulse pressure – PP) and area under the systolic portion of the waveform (AUC) are intimately linked to SV, vascular compliance and systemic vascular resistance. Under steady-state conditions, when vascular compliance and resistance are relatively constant, SV becomes the main determinant of PP and AUC. If CO is measured directly under these static conditions using indicator or temperature dilution techniques then a mathematical relationship can be established linking PP, AUC and SV. This indirect estimation of CO using parameters such as PP and AUC obtained from arterial waveforms is known as 'arterial pulse contour analysis'.
- Requires insertion of an arterial line (special femoral arterial line required for PiCCO).
- Physiological and therapeutic changes in vessel wall diameter are assumed to reflect changes in cardiac performance – this effect is minimised by intermittent calibration.

- PiCCO device is calibrated via a transpulmonary thermodilution technique.
- LiDCO device is calibrated via a lithium dilution technique.
- PiCCO device identifies AUC by recognising the dicrotic notch on the arterial waveform and this is used to determine SV. It is converted to an absolute number by calibration. In addition to CO and SV, PiCCO device also provides 'dynamic' indicators of volume responsiveness: stroke volume variation (SVV), pulse pressure variation (PPV), systolic pressure variation (SPV) as well as a number of volumetric markers of preload: global end-diastolic volume, intrathoracic blood volume and extravascular lung water.
- LiDCO utilises an existing arterial line and tracks the power of the arterial waveform rather than the contour in order to track changes in SV. Theoretical advantage of LiDCO is the reduction of the effect of reflected waves because the device does not need to identify specific parts of the arterial waveform. It also provides dynamic indicators of preload (SVV, SPV and PPV). LiDCO calibration is not possible in the presence of atracurium.
- Relatively minimally invasive systems, providing continuous beat-to-beat monitoring.
- Can be used in awake patients.
- Both are not reliable with arrhythmias.

71. DEPTH OF ANAESTHESIA MONITORING

The definitions and management of awareness are dealt with in Study Guide 2, Part 3, 'Critical Incidents', Chapter 53, 'Awareness'.

Depth of anaesthesia (DOA) monitoring can be used to reduce the risk of accidental awareness during general anaesthesia and to titrate the dose of anaesthetic agent used in order to minimise the adverse effects of excessively deep anaesthesia (hypotension, impaired cardiac function, increased nausea and vomiting, and delayed recovery), which would also have cost-saving benefits. NICE in 2012 recommended the use of electroencephalography (EEG)-based DOA monitoring (Bispectral Index (BIS), E-Entropy or Narcotrend-Compact M) as an 'option' during any type of general anaesthesia where patients were deemed to be at 'higher risk' of awareness or excessive DOA and in patients receiving total intravenous anaesthesia. The National Audit Project 5 published in 2014 found that DOA monitoring was only used in 2.83% of general anaesthetics administered in the UK.

How can the depth of anaesthesia be monitored?

Electroencephalography-based monitors:

EEG-based DOA monitors use electrodes on the forehead to measure the EEG activity, which is then processed using various algorithms that are currently a commercial secret. Propofol, thiopentone and volatile anaesthetic agents all produce a similar pattern of EEG changes with increasing brain concentrations and corresponding DOA (↑ high-frequency EEG components – ↑ low-frequency EEG components – ↑ waveform amplitude – ↑ regularity of EEG signal – burst suppression with deep anaesthesia – isoelectric 'flat line' EEG with very deep anaesthesia). Ketamine, nitrous oxide and xenon do not produce this same pattern of EEG changes and therefore the use of EEG-derived indices to guide anaesthetic administration becomes less useful if these agents are among the anaesthetic drugs being used.

> **BIS monitor** – this is currently the most commonly used technique. A disposable four-electrode sensor is placed on the patient's forehead and cortical EEG activity is recorded. A proprietary algorithm processes this data and produces a dimensionless number between 0 and 100, which provides a measure of the DOA. When the patient is awake,

cerebrocortical activity is increased with more higher-frequency signals generated. This leads to the generation of a higher number:

- 0–40 Burst suppression (0 = 'flat-line' or electrical silence)
- 40–60 Surgical anaesthesia where auditory processing and reflex movement are still possible but memory is less likely – low probability of explicit recall
- 60–85 Increasing sedation, impaired memory processing but arousable with stimulation
- 85–100 Awake and capable of explicit recall.

The B-Aware trial published in 2004 compared BIS-guided anaesthesia with standard care in 2463 adult patients with neuromuscular blockade who were at increased risk of awareness. The results indicated a lower incidence of accidental awareness in the BIS group compared with the standard care group.

> **E-Entropy monitors** – this measures the irregularity in spontaneous brain and facial muscular activity using a disposable three-electrode sensor placed on the patient's forehead. It uses a proprietary algorithm to process EEG and frontal electromyography data to produce two values that indicate the DOA-response entropy (RE) and state entropy (SE). Highly irregular signals with variation of wavelength and amplitude over time produce high entropy values and may indicate that the patient is awake or aware. More ordered signals with less variation produce low or zero entropy values, indicating suppression of brain electrical activity. The RE scale ranges from 0 (no brain activity) to 100 (fully awake) and the SE scale ranges from 0 to 91. The target range is 40–60. RE and SE values near 40 indicate a low probability of awareness with explicit recall.

> **Power spectral analysis (PSA)** – this is also based on EEG analysis. The raw EEG data undergo Fourier's analysis to break it down into its constituent sine waves. These are then processed and displayed graphically. The 'power' wave amplitude drops as the DOA increases. There are problems with inter-patient variability.

> **Auditory-evoked potentials (AEP)** – this has evolved on the basis that the auditory sense disappears last when undergoing anaesthesia. A series of clicks is delivered into the patient's ear as they are anaesthetised. The resulting EEG is monitored and analysed to give an AEP index (AEP > 80 is awake and AEP < 50 is asleep). Unlike BIS monitoring, the system exhibits much less hysteresis and there are defined 'awake' and 'asleep' points. It is now being marketed with an algorithm giving arbitrary values of 0–100.

> **Raw EEG** – this can be accurate but needs expert interpretation.

Clinical methods:

> **Clinical signs** – in the spontaneously ventilating patient, movement and the depth and frequency of respiration are useful indicators of anaesthetic adequacy. In the paralysed patient these features are lost and instead signs of sympathetic stimulation are often used. The PRST (or Evan's) scoring system (pressure, rate, sweating and tears) was developed to provide an objective assessment of sympathetic stimulation. However, indirect autonomic or involuntary responses have all proved to be unreliable signs of consciousness. These scoring systems are not specific to the effects of anaesthesia and absence of sympathetic activity does not exclude awareness (in fact, there is good evidence from large case series that autonomic responses are uncommon in cases of reported accidental awareness under anaesthesia).

> **Isolated forearm technique** – a tourniquet is applied to the arm and inflated to above arterial blood pressure before a neuromuscular blocking drug is administered through a vein elsewhere in the body. Therefore, the muscle relaxant does not reach the muscles of the arm distal to the tourniquet and movement of the hand is preserved. If the patient is aware, they will be able to move their hand to alert the anaesthetist. Tunstall, an obstetric anaesthetist, originally described the technique in 1977, but very few anaesthetists actually use this technique today.

> **Lower oesophageal contractility** – a balloon catheter with a distal pressure transducer is placed in the lower oesophagus. Provoked oesophageal contractions are triggered by inflation of the balloon while spontaneous oesophageal contractions are triggered by stress and emotion in an awake patient. These contractions are recorded by the pressure transducer, and using an algorithm, the device generates the oesophageal contractility index for that patient.

Other methods:

> **End-tidal anaesthetic gas monitoring:** National Audit Project (NAP) 5 identified that end-tidal anaesthetic gas monitoring used with audible alarms appropriately set was a reliable way of ensuring a desired concentration of inhalational agent was given to a patient. The B-Unaware trial published in 2008 and the BAG-RECALL trial in 2011 compared BIS-guided anaesthesia with a protocol in which alarms were used to alert the anaesthetist to keep end-tidal anaesthetic gases at an age-adjusted MAC >0.7. These trials found no difference in risk of awareness between the two groups.

What are some of the limitations in EEG-based monitoring of depth of anaesthesia?

There is considerable heterogeneity and uncertainty between various studies using EEG-based monitors to determine DOA. This is mainly due to the individual response to anaesthesia, diverse case mix and the variation in administering anaesthesia in clinical practice. It is also not fully established how EEG DOA monitors perform when drugs such as ketamine or nitrous oxide are used in conjunction with propofol or inhalation anaesthetic agents.

In what other settings might a BIS monitor be used?

On intensive care units, BIS can be used to monitor burst suppression, which is a technique used to reduce cerebral metabolic oxygen requirements in patients with head injuries and raised intracranial pressures or in status epilepticus. It can also be used to reduce awareness in those paralysed for long time.

72. SAFETY FEATURES OF THE ANAESTHETIC MACHINE

Despite the advances in technology and the development of newer and more sophisticated anaesthetic machines, it is still an essential requirement to understand the safety features governing the use of such devices.

What are the principal functions of the anaesthetic machine?

> To receive compressed gases from their supplies (pipeline or cylinder)
> To accurately and continuously deliver a gas and volatile mixture of the desired composition
> To avoid delivering hypoxic gas mixtures
> To deliver a gas mixture to the patient at a safe pressure (to avoid barotrauma)

What are the safety features of an anaesthetic machine?

One of the most important safety features is the presence of a trained, competent anaesthetist and a serviced and checked anaesthetic machine. A pre-use check to ensure the correct functioning of the anaesthetic machine and equipment is essential to patient safety. The importance of this check is recognised internationally and is included in the World Health Organization Safer Surgical Checklist. Prior to commencing any anaesthetic, it is essential to have a self-inflating bag, an alternative source of oxygen (e.g. a cylinder), relevant airway equipment and emergency drugs immediately available.

The anaesthetic machine itself has numerous safety features built in and in order not to miss anything, it is best to breakdown the anaesthetic machine into systems and work your way from the back of the anaesthetic machine to the common gas outlet.

Power supply and battery back-up
> Modern anaesthetic machines have visual and audible indicators to alert the anaesthetist of a power failure.
> A back-up, re-chargeable battery is present, and this must be checked as part of the Association of Anaesthetists of Great Britain and Ireland (AAGBI) anaesthetic machine check to ensure it is charged.

Gas supplies
> Pipeline – colour-coded, flexible hosepipes (black = air, white = oxygen and blue = nitrous oxide) connect to the wall via a Schrader valve (gas specific and non-interchangeable) and connect to the back of the anaesthetic machine via non-interchangeable screw threads (NIST – gas specific and permanently fixed).

> Cylinders – colour-coded gas cylinders (oxygen = black body with white shoulder, nitrous oxide = blue body with blue shoulder and air = black body with white and black shoulders) act as an emergency source of gases should primary piped gas delivery fail. They connect to the back of the anaesthetic machine via a pin-indexed system (oxygen = 2.5, nitrous oxide = 3.5 and air = 1.5) incorporating a Bodok seal to make the connection gas-tight. They are now made of molybdenum steel, which is lighter and stronger than its carbon steel predecessor.
> Pressure regulators reduce the pressure of cylinder gases to approximately $400\,kP_a$ (i.e. the same as piped gas pressure), thereby protecting the anaesthetic machine from damage due to high gas pressures.
> Pipeline and gas cylinder pressure indicators (traditional machines used a Bourdon gauge).

Gas flow measurement and control

> Flow control needle valves govern the transition from high- to low-pressure systems, reducing the pressure from 4 bar to just above atmospheric pressure as gas enters the flowmeter block.
> Flowmeters can be mechanical or electronic.
>   • Mechanical – rotameters are the conventional mechanical flowmeter. They are constant pressure, variable orifice flowmeters, which allow fresh gas flow rates to be regulated and measured (calibrated to individual gases as the density and viscosity of the gases are important). Oxygen is the last gas to be added to the fresh gas flow, which prevents delivery of a hypoxic gas mixture should a proximal crack in the flowmeter occur. Rotameters are produced with anti-static material to prevent the bobbin 'sticking', which could result in inaccurate fresh gas flow measurement. The control knobs are labelled and colour-coded. The oxygen control knob is larger, protrudes further and is grooved to allow differentiation from the air and nitrous oxide control knobs.
>   • Electronic – modern anaesthetic machines use microprocessors to control gas flow and the flow is indicated either electronically by a numerical display or using virtual flow tubes. There is a pneumatic back-up in the event of a power failure, which continues the delivery of fresh gas. Some systems allow low flow rates (<500 mL/min) to be utilised, reducing cost and pollution.
> Anti-hypoxic mixture devices prevent the inadvertent delivery of a hypoxic-inspired gas mixture, and they can be mechanical, pneumatic or electronic.
>   • Mechanical devices use a chain to link the nitrous oxide flow to a minimum oxygen flow.
>   • Pneumatic devices use a ratio mixer valve.
>   • Electronic devices use a paramagnetic oxygen analyser to continuously sample the gas mixtures from the flowmeters.

Vaporisers

> They sit on the back bar of the anaesthetic machine and convert volatile liquid into vapour and add a controlled amount of volatile to the fresh gas flow. The common manifold systems that prevent the use of more than one vaporiser at any time are the Selectatec type (Ohmeda) and the Interlock type (Drager).

> They are colour-coded (blue = desflurane, yellow = sevoflurane and purple = isoflurane) and have a liquid-level indicator. The modern devices have a non-spill reservoir allowing up to 180 ° of tilt.
> Filling devices are geometrically coded and agent specific, designed to prevent incorrect vaporiser filling.
> Back-bar pressure relief valves are situated downstream of the vaporisers and vent off gas mixtures at pressures greater than $35\,kP_a$. This prevents barotrauma to the flow meters and vaporisers but not the patient.

Oxygen failure warning device

> British standards specify that the alarm should be powered solely by the oxygen supply pressure. It is activated when the oxygen supply pressure falls below 2 bar and when this has occurred flow of all other gases ceases and atmospheric air is entrained. The alarm produces a sound of at least 60 dB for a minimum 7 seconds.

Oxygen flush

> 100% oxygen is supplied from the high-pressure circuit upstream, bypassing flowmeters and vaporisers, and is delivered at rates between 35 and 75 L/min and a pressure of about $400\,kP_a$.
> There is a risk of barotrauma and of anaesthetic agent dilution with its use.

Adjustable pressure-limiting valve

> Allows excess gas to escape when a preset pressure is exceeded, thereby reducing risk of barotrauma to the patient.

Common gas outlet

> Standardised 22 mm male outer diameter/15 mm female internal diameter connection accommodating only breathing system attachments (circle or T-piece).

Monitoring

> Monitors have now become integrated within modern anaesthetic machines. Oxygen, inhalation agent and end-tidal carbon dioxide concentration analysers, gas volume and airway pressure measurements are all essential and are monitored and displayed on LED screens.
> Prioritised preset alarms with audible and visual components exist. Alarm limits can also be individualised and the monitor settings can be changed (e.g. local anaesthesia, cardiopulmonary bypass or to detect pacing spikes).

73. DISCONNECTION MONITORS

Which monitors are essential for the induction and maintenance of general anaesthesia?	> Trained anaesthetist > Anaesthetic machine that has been checked, airway equipment, emergency drugs, self-inflating bag and alternative oxygen supply to be immediately available > ECG, blood pressure and oxygen saturations > F_iO_2, E_tCO_2 with capnography and inhalational agent concentration ($\pm$MAC) > Ventilating volumes and airway pressures > Temperature monitoring and peripheral nerve stimulation if muscle relaxant used > Depth of anaesthesia monitoring (e.g BIS or entropy) if total intravenous anaesthesia or muscle relaxant used

Which monitors would alert you to a disconnection in the breathing circuit?	> The vigilant anaesthetist is the most important monitor!
	> In order to know which monitors would alarm, three important factors must be considered:
	  • Where in the circuit has the disconnection taken place
	  • Whether the patient is breathing spontaneously or being ventilated
	  • What alarm parameters have been set
	> Point of disconnection – working from the patient end to the anaesthetic machine, a disconnection in the breathing circuit can occur between:
	  • The catheter mount and the airway device
	  • The HME filter and the catheter mount
	  • The breathing circuit and the HME filter
	  • The anaesthetic machine and the breathing circuit
	> Spontaneously breathing – working from the machine end to the patient, if the disconnection has occurred proximal to the point at which $EtCO_2$ sampling takes place (i.e. the $EtCO_2$ sampling line is still connected and in continuity with the patient) then an $EtCO_2$ trace would still be present but the patient would not be receiving fresh gas flow with inhalation agents from the anaesthetic machine. Inspired oxygen concentration and volatile concentrations would remain unaffected but the corresponding expired concentrations would be zero.
	> Ventilated patient – whether the disconnection occurs proximal or distal to the $EtCO_2$ sampling port is irrelevant as the patient is apnoeic. The $EtCO_2$ measurement and trace would be lost, tidal volumes and minute ventilation would fall, and airway pressures would drop triggering alarms (provided they have not been switched off). The ventilator would also alarm as the bellows would not be able to fill. Expired inhalational agent concentration, MAC and expired oxygen concentrations would also drop.

What would be the potential consequences of a disconnection in the breathing circuit?

> If disconnection occurs in the presence of a trained, vigilant anaesthetist, then theoretically it should be identified rapidly with no significant consequences.

> However, if it takes longer to identify, then a spontaneously breathing patient would continue to breathe room air and over time would wake up (provided he or she were not receiving total intravenous anaesthesia).

> A ventilated patient, following a disconnection, would remain apnoeic, oxygen saturations would fall (the time at which this occurs would depend on the original FiO_2 the patient was receiving), would become hypoxic and, if not corrected, there would be associated ECG changes (most likely bradycardia), hypotension and eventually the patient would suffer a cardiac arrest. Therefore, depending on the outcome of the disconnection, this event could be classified as a critical incident or a serious incident requiring investigation (SIRI).

74. BREATHING SYSTEMS

A question on breathing systems often starts with the examiner showing photographs of different types of systems, asking you to identify them and explain how they function.

There are three main objectives when using a breathing system:
> *To supply O_2 to the patient*
> *To allow removal of CO_2 from the system and avoid rebreathing*
> *To supply anaesthetic gases to the patient*

There are several classification systems, but the most commonly used (and examined) is the Mapleson classification system (Professor Bill Mapleson worked in Cardiff and classified the breathing systems in 1954).

Describe the movement of gas within each system.

The respiratory cycle comprises three phases: inspiration, expiration and the expiratory pause.
> During inspiration, gas is drawn in from the equipment.
> In quiet breathing, the average 70 kg patient's tidal volume is approximately 500 mL. At 20 breaths per minute, their minute volume (MV) would be 10 L/min. In order to avoid rebreathing, the fresh gas flow rate would have to exceed the patient's MV. This would result in very high volumes of gas needing to be delivered. This is wasteful and requires high flow rates that would be uncomfortable for the patient.
> With maximum effort, the average 70 kg patient can draw in approximately 5 L of gas over about 2 seconds. Again, unless flow rates were extremely high the patient would entrain air.
> To overcome these problems, reservoir bags have been added to the breathing systems.
> During deep inspiration the patient can draw oxygen and gases from these as well as from the fresh gas flow.
> At the beginning of expiration, gas expired is from the anatomical dead space, so it does not contain CO_2 and is not depleted of O_2. This gas is fit to be inhaled again.
> As expiration continues, alveolar gas is exhaled next, this contains CO_2 and is O_2 deplete. It is desirable to rid the system of this gas before the next inspiration.
> Adjustable pressure-relieving (APL) valves have been added to some circuits to vent waste gases and overcome the problem of rebreathing.

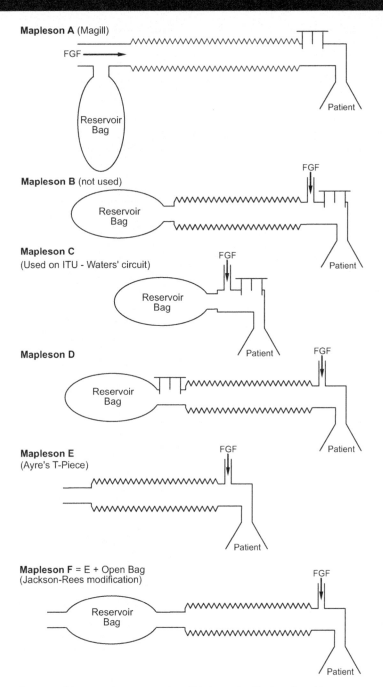

Fig. 74.1 Diagrammatic respresentation of Mapleson classification of breathing systems

Mapleson A (non-co-axial 'Magill' system)
Spontaneous ventilation

When describing breathing systems always start with the statement, 'The patient has just exhaled, the equipment is full of fresh gas and I put the mask over the patient's face. At the perfect flow rate ...'

> The patient inhales fresh gas, from the supply and from the reservoir bag, which deflates proportionally.
> The patient exhales and the dead space volume is expelled into the breathing system, passing down the tubing and fills the reservoir bag again. In addition, the fresh gas flow will also contribute to filling the bag.

> After the dead space gas, the alveolar gas is exhaled. At this stage the reservoir bag is already filled and so the pressure in the system begins to rise. Because of this, the alveolar gas is vented through the APL valve and lost from the system, so avoiding rebreathing.
> If the fresh gas flow is too low, the bag will not be filled solely by dead space gas. Some alveolar gas will be able to enter the bag, and the patient will rebreathe.
> If the fresh gas flow is too high, the fresh gas flow will fill the bag to a degree and dead space gas will be vented along with alveolar gas. While this avoids rebreathing, it is wasteful and inefficient.

Controlled ventilation

> The anaesthetist squeezes the bag, forcing gas into the patient. Some gas, however, will be vented from the expiratory valve near the patient. At the end of inspiration, the reservoir bag will not be full.
> During exhalation, dead space and alveolar gas will move down to fill the reservoir bag.

Unless the gas flows are high, 2.5 × MV, rebreathing will occur.
The Mapleson A is:

> Efficient in spontaneous ventilation (70 mL/kg/min)
> Inefficient for controlled ventilation (2.5 × MV).

Mapleson A (co-axial version 'Lack' system)
Co-axial means there is an inner tube surrounded by an outer one.

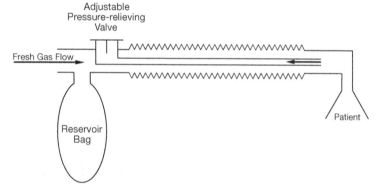

Fig. 74.2 Co-axial Mapleson A

The Lack is a version of the Mapleson A, which was designed to move the pressure release valve away from the patient and so make it less awkward and bulky to use. The fresh gas flows down the outside tubing, and gas is vented via the inner tubing. The reservoir bag is in the inspiratory limb, while the pressure release valve is in the expiratory limb. The gas flows required in the system are the same as for the standard A. The Lack is bulkier than the Bain (see next page) because the inner tube has to have a sufficiently large diameter to minimise expiratory resistance.

Mapleson B and C
These are essentially the same, but the C has shorter tubing. The B is not used. The C is used for transfer, or 'bagging' patients on ICU. This system needs high gas flows to prevent rebreathing (2.5 × MV for spontaneous and controlled ventilation).

The Mapleson C is colloquially referred to as a 'Waters' circuit', though strictly this is inaccurate as a true Waters' circuit would include a canister of soda lime to absorb CO_2 and prevent rebreathing. These are not manufactured any more.

Mapleson D (non-co-axial system)
Spontaneous ventilation

The patient has just exhaled, the equipment is full of fresh gas and I put the mask over the patient's face. At the perfect flow rate:

> The patient inhales fresh gas, from the supply and from the reservoir bag, which deflates proportionally
> The patient exhales and the dead space volume is expelled into the breathing system. The fresh gas flow and the exhaled dead space gas mix and both pass down the tubing to fill the reservoir bag
> After the dead space gas, the alveolar gas is exhaled. At this stage the reservoir bag is already filled and so the pressure in the system begins to rise. Because of this, the alveolar gas is vented through the pressure release valve and lost from the system so avoiding rebreathing
> During the expiratory pause, fresh gas continues to push exhaled alveolar gas down towards the reservoir bag (as the pressure release valve is further away than in the A) and rebreathing will occur at gas flows of $<2.5 \times MV$.

Controlled ventilation

> The patient exhales and a mixture of fresh gas and dead space gas enters the bag, as described above.
> The anaesthetist squeezes the bag and fresh gas from the distal tubing is forced into the patient and a variable amount of gas from the reservoir enters the patient. Following this, the pressure in the system rises (according to the patient's lung compliance) and further gas gets vented from the expiratory valve.

The Mapleson D is:

> Inefficient for spontaneous ventilation ($2.5 \times MV$)
> Efficient for controlled ventilation (70 mL/kg/min).

Mapleson D (co-axial 'Bain' system)

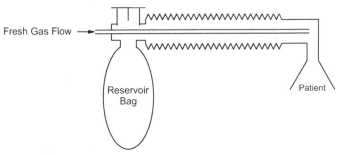

Fig. 74.3 Co-axial Mapleson D

In this circuit the fresh gas flows down the inner tubing, and exhaled gas enters the outer tubing. Both the reservoir bag and APL valve are in the expiratory limb. The Bain is equally efficient for controlled or spontaneous ventilation.

During controlled ventilation at a flow rate of 70 mL/kg/min, the patient will in fact be rebreathing. However, because we tend to over-ventilate our patients, their end tidal CO_2 will not actually rise despite the fact they are rebreathing. If we managed not to over-ventilate, we would actually see a rising E_TCO_2 as evidence of this. To truly avoid rebreathing during controlled ventilation in the Bain circuit, we would need to use $2.5 \times MV$, the same flow rate as is necessary to avoid it in spontaneous ventilation.

Mapleson E

This is also called the Ayre's T-piece after the man who invented it.

It has no valves or reservoir bag and so is a very low resistance system. This makes it suitable for use in paediatrics.

Mapleson F

This is an E with the 'Jackson–Rees modification': an open-ended reservoir bag connected to the end of the tubing. This allows for the application of CPAP and controlled ventilation.

In both E and F, fresh gas flows of 2.5 × MV are required to prevent rebreathing.

Table 74.1 Volume of fresh gas flow required to prevent rebreathing during spontaneous and controlled ventilation using the Mapleson breathing systems

Mapleson classification	Spontaneous ventilation	Controlled ventilation
A	70 mL/kg/min	2.5 × MV
B	2.5 × MV	2.5 × MV
C	2.5 × MV	2.5 × MV
D	2.5 × MV	70 mL/kg/min
E	2.5 × MV	2.5 × MV
< 20 kg	2.5 × MV (minimum 3 L/min)	1000 mL + 100 mL/kg/min

75. RESUSCITATION BAGS AND VALVES

Questions about this equipment will revolve around non-rebreathing valves, so it is essential to be able to name, describe and even draw the various types.

What type of resuscitation bag do you find on a cardiac arrest trolley?

A self-inflating bag with a non-rebreathing valve and mask is found on a cardiac arrest trolley. This is a compact and portable ventilating system that does not require a pressurised gas supply to work. It consists of a fresh gas inlet with a one-way valve (commonly in communication with an O_2 reservoir bag to increase FiO_2), an entrainment valve at the inlet (to allow entrainment of air if oxygen supply does not meet respiratory demands), a self-inflating bag (1500 mL for adults, 500 mL for children and 250 mL for infants), a non-rebreathing valve and a pressure-relieving valve to prevent barotrauma.

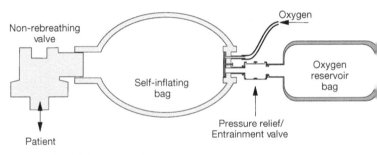

Fig. 75.1 Self-inflating resuscitation bag

How does it work?

The main component in a self-inflating resuscitation bag is the non-rebreathing valve (e.g. Reuben, Ambu E or Laerdal valves). Their function is to ensure that gas flows out of the self-inflating bag and into the patient during inspiration and that exhaled gases pass out through the expiratory port and do not re-enter the self-inflating bag.

Non-rebreathing valves are made up of the following:
> Inspiratory port, often coloured blue ('blue to bag'), supplying fresh gas for inspiration.
> Expiratory port, often coloured yellow or gold ('gold for go'), allowing the exit of exhaled gases.
> Patient port that connects to the airway adjunct (mask, LMA, OETT).
> One-way valve or valves ensuring exhaled gases are not rebreathed.

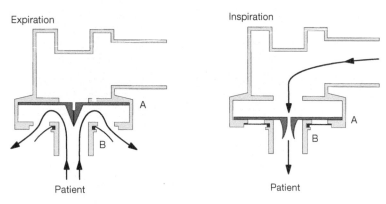

Fig. 75.2   Non-rebreathe valve

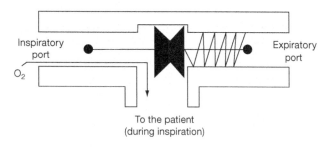

To the patient
(during inspiration)

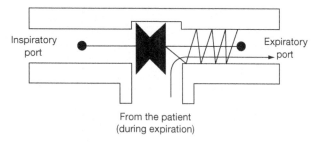

From the patient
(during expiration)

Fig. 75.3   Reuben valve

Reuben valve:

> This consists of a spring-loaded bobbin.
> During positive pressure ventilation, as the bag is squeezed, the bobbin is pushed across and closes the expiratory port, allowing fresh gas to enter the patient.
> During expiration, as the bag relaxes, the bobbin shifts to the opposite side and closes the inspiratory port, allowing exhaled gases to escape through the expiratory port.
> The bag then self-inflates, drawing in air from the room and oxygen from the reservoir bag ready to deliver the next breath.
> The valve can jam, keeping the inspiratory port continuously open, which risks hyperinflating the lungs.
> The valves offer resistance (0.8 cm H_2O during inspiration and 1 cm H_2O during expiration) and therefore can significantly increase the work of breathing and impair passive expiration in the spontaneously ventilating patient. Therefore, these devices should be used cautiously in patients with respiratory fatigue ('assisted' breaths should be given to such patients by gently squeezing the bag when they inspire, which helps open the valves, thereby reducing resistance).

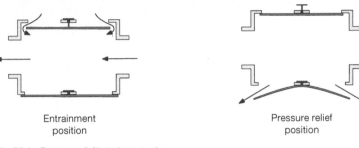

Entrainment
position

Pressure relief
position

Fig. 75.4 Pressure relief/entrainment valve

Ambu E valve:

> This is a double-leaf valve.
> During positive pressure ventilation, the inspiratory port leaf valve is pushed across and seals the expiratory port, thereby allowing gases to enter the patient.
> During expiration, the inspiratory port leaf valve gets pushed back, sealing the inspiratory port while the expiratory port leaf valve gets forced open, allowing exhaled gases to escape into the atmosphere.
> During low inspiratory gas flow rates, the inspiratory port leaf valve may not give a good seal across the expiratory port and hence some of the fresh gas can escape across the valve, reducing the fresh gas supply to the patient.
> The valve offers resistance and should be used cautiously in the spontaneously ventilating patient.

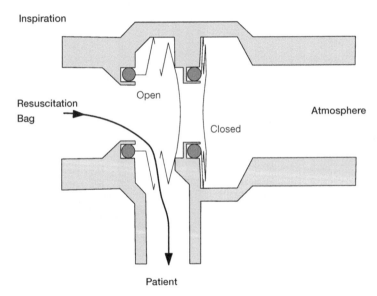

Fig. 75.5 Ambu E valve during inspiration

Expiration

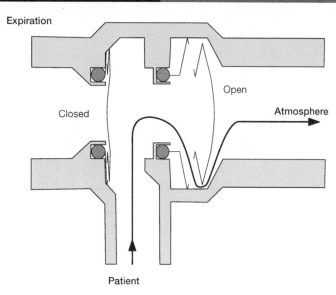

Fig. 75.6 Ambu E valve during expiration

Principle of the Ambu 'mushroom' valve

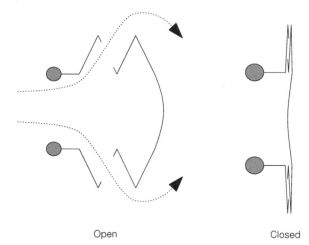

Open   Closed

Fig. 75.7 Principle of Ambu mushroom valve

What factors determine the oxygen concentration that can be delivered to the patient?

> FiO_2
> Oxygen flow rate
> Reservoir bag volume (adult size approximately 2600 mL)
> Inspiratory flow rate
> Respiratory rate
> Valve type

76. VENTILATORS

How can ventilators be classified?

A question on ventilators will often follow on from a physics question about flow. The simplest way to address this question is to classify ventilation according to the Mapleson classification, which separates it into either 'pressure-generated' or 'flow-generated' ventilation.

A ventilator is a device that delivers gas to the lungs

Pressure Generator

- Delivers gas to the patient at a **constant inspiratory pressure** set by the operator.

- Usually **time cycled** (i.e. the operator sets the pressure, the number of breaths per minute and the inspiratory:expiratory time ratio and the machine will deliver breaths accordingly).

- Inspiratory flow rates and tidal volume achieved will depend on the patient's lung compliance (i.e. the stiffer the lungs the lower the resulting tidal volume delivered).

- Risk of barotrauma is low.

- Risk of volutrauma is higher (so set volume limits).

- The system has some ability to compensate for leaks, as it always acts to deliver a preset pressure for a set amount of time.

Flow Generator

- Delivers gas to patient at a **constant inspiratory flow rate** until it has delivered a pre-set tidal volume.

- Cycles when the **set tidal volume** has been delivered (i.e. the operator sets the volume to be delivered, the number of breaths and the I:E ratio).

- Inspiratory pressures reached depend on the patient's lung compliance (i.e. the lower the compliance, the higher the peak inspiration pressure).

- Higher risk of barotrauma (so set pressure limits).

- Lower risk of volutrauma.

- Any leak in the circuit is not compensated for, as the ventilator will perceive that the lost volume has been delivered to the patient.

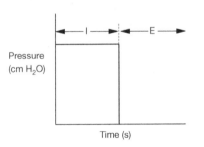

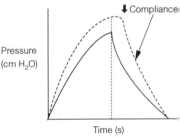

Graphs comparing pressure profiles of the two different ventilation modes

Fig. 76.1 Comparison of pressure vs. flow ventilation

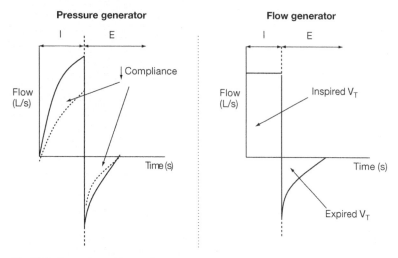

Fig. 76.2 Comparison of flow profiles for pressure-generated and flow-generated ventilators

A third type of ventilator is called the high-frequency oscillating ventilator (HFOV).

HFOV employs an 'open lung' strategy, using high PEEP and very small tidal volumes (1–3 mL/kg) at respiratory rates of up to 15 Hz (i.e. 900 breaths per minute!).

It aims to reduce distending pressures in poorly compliant lungs (e.g. in ARDS) and is recommended for those patients requiring a high FiO_2 >0.60 and with high mean airways pressures >24 cm H_2O.

The mechanism of oxygenation with this type of ventilation is not fully understood, but diffusion, convection and Pendelluft (i.e. movement of gas between different alveolar units with different time constants) are thought to play a part.

DEFINITIONS OF VENTILATORY MODES

CPAP – Continuous Positive Airway Pressure

- A positive pressure (cm H_2O) is applied to the airway of a spontaneously breathing patient via a facial or nasal mask. The pressure is constant through all phases of the ventilatory cycle.
- The positive pressure helps to prevent alveolar and airway closure during expiration and improves lung compliance by moving the lungs up the compliance curve.
- This mode of ventilation is used in the treatment of obstructive sleep apnoea.

PEEP – Positive End Expiratory Pressure

- This is very similar to CPAP, except that it applies to mechanically ventilated patients.
- PEEP is a set level of pressure (cm H_2O) below which the circuit is not allowed to fall at the end of expiration. It is usually set between 5 and 10 cm H_2O.
- It helps to prevent alveolar and airway closure during expiration and improves lung compliance by moving the lungs up the compliance curve.

BiPAP – Bi-level Positive Airway Pressure

- This is a trade name of a particular make of non-invasive ventilators.
- BiPAP is given via a face mask, usually to a conscious and spontaneously ventilating patient.
- The operator sets two levels of pressure; the first is effectively the PEEP, i.e. the level below which the circuit is not allowed to fall. The second is the positive inspiratory pressure, which the ventilator delivers to the patient.
- The machine senses when the patient is taking a breath (via a pressure transducer which senses negative pressure in the system) and then augments their breath to the set pressure. In most cases, cycling is controlled by the machine sensing the patient's respiratory effort. Some models can deliver time-cycled positive pressure if the patient fails to make any respiratory effort after a set time has elapsed.

PC – Pressure Control

- Pressure control is used in a mechanically ventilated patient. It is the most basic mode of ventilation.
- The operator sets either the desired tidal volume or desired pressure and the number of breaths per minute, and the ventilator will deliver these.
- Any respiratory effort that the patient makes is 'ignored' by the ventilator.

PS – Pressure Support

- Pressure support is used for weaning patients from the ventilator.
- As in BiPAP, the ventilator senses the patient's inspiratory effort and augments it with a pre-set inspiratory pressure.
- It is usual to set two levels of pressure, the principle being the same as that described above for BiPAP.

SIMV – Synchronised Intermittent Mandatory Ventilation

- This mode is a 'half-way house' between PC and PS.
- The operator sets the desired tidal volume or inspiratory pressure and the number of breaths per minute. The ventilator will then deliver these breaths.
- However, if the patient makes an inspiratory effort the machine will sense this and augment their breath.

PRVC – Pressure Regulated Volume Control

- In this mode, the operator sets the tidal volume and the machine will deliver this volume in such a way as to give the lowest resultant inspiratory pressure.
- This mode has been developed to try to reduce the risk of barotrauma and to address the issue of different areas of the lung having different compliance in lung diseases such as ARDS.

77. VAPORISERS

Classify the types of vaporiser in use.

A vaporiser is a device used during inhalational anaesthesia to administer a given concentration of a volatile anaesthetic agent. There are various types on the market and they can be classified as follows:

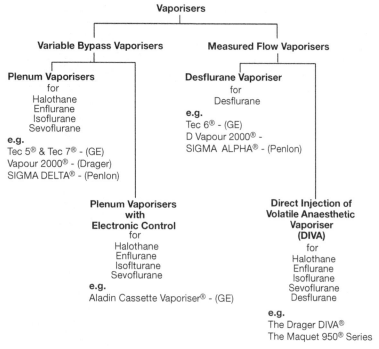

Fig. 77.1   Classification of vaporisers

How do variable bypass plenum vaporisers work?

Variable bypass vaporisers work as the name suggests. There are two possible paths for fresh gas to flow through the vaporiser: via the vaporising chamber itself or via the bypass pathway. Gas, which enters the vaporising chamber, becomes fully saturated with vapour. As it exits the vaporiser it is reintroduced to the vapour-free bypass gas and the two mix. This mixture is then delivered to the patient. The resulting concentration of volatile agent present in the mixture depends on how much fresh gas went through each of the pathways.

The path of the fresh gas flow is determined by the 'splitting valve', which is attached to the control dial on the outside of the vaporiser. This dial is calibrated from 0 to 5% for isoflurane and 0 to 8% for sevoflurane. When it is turned to zero, the valve is closed and no fresh gas flows through the vaporising chamber. As the anaesthetist turns the control dial to deliver a higher concentration of volatile, the splitting valve opens wider, allowing a greater proportion of the fresh gas flow to travel though the volatile chamber. The ratio of fresh gas flowing through the chamber to that flowing via the bypass pathway is called the 'splitting ratio'.

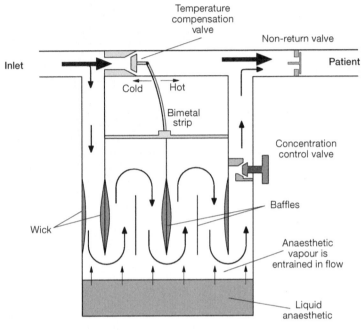

Fig. 77.2   Variable bypass (plenum) vaporiser

What are the potential problems with this device and how are they overcome?

Problem	A **high fresh gas flow** through the vaporiser could affect its output because it may result in insufficient vapour being available to fully saturate the fresh gas passing through the chamber.
Solution	Inside the vaporising chamber a series of wicks and baffles are dipped into the volatile liquid. This greatly increases the surface area of volatile anaesthetic exposed to fresh gas flow, ensuring that the gas leaves the chamber fully saturated. In this way, the output concentration is independent of flow.

Chapter 62

Problem	As an anaesthetic liquid turns to vapour it absorbs energy (the latent heat of fusion – *see* Chapter 62, 'States of matter'). Consequently, there is a fall in the **temperature** of the liquid in the chamber, which leads to a decrease in the rate of vaporisation because fewer molecules will have sufficient energy to evaporate. This leads to a fall in the SVP of the volatile and so to a fall in the concentration of anaesthetic agent delivered to the patient. This effect is more marked at high flow rates when the rate of vaporisation increases.
Solution	Plenum vaporisers are not electrically heated however, their casing contains copper, which is a very good conductor of heat from the environment and so conducts energy to the liquid as it cools, helping to mitigate this effect.
	The addition of a 'bimetallic strip' helps to compensate for fluctuations in output due to temperature. As the chamber cools, the two different metals comprising the strip contract to different degrees and cause the strip to bend. This increases the splitting ratio of the free gas flow as the temperature drops and vice versa.

Problem	The **'pumping effect'**. Positive pressure ventilation of the patient will cause intermittent pressure changes, both upstream to the patient (desirable) and downstream to the vaporiser (undesirable). If positive pressure is transmitted to the vaporiser chamber, it can result in gas saturated with vapour being displaced 'backwards' and into the bypass channel. As the positive pressure is released, there will be an expansion of gas forward towards the patient. When the vapour from the usually vapour-free bypass channel mixes with the fully saturated gas from the vaporiser chamber it will result in an increase in the concentration of anaesthetic agent delivered to the patient.
Solution	A non-return valve is inserted at the outlet of the vaporiser.
	The vaporiser is designed to have a high internal resistance, to resist the changes in flow caused by positive pressure ventilation.
Problem	**Incorrect anaesthetic** liquid introduced to vaporiser.
Solution	Standardised colour coding of vaporisers and bottles (sevoflurane – yellow, isoflurane – purple, desflurane – blue), and keyed fillers reduce this risk.
Problem	**Over-filling** can cause overdose and spillage of anaesthetic liquid onto the patient circuit is potentially fatal.
Solution	Low filling ports help to reduce the risk of overfilling. Transparent window with a 'fill line' is visible on the front of the vaporiser.
Problem	**Tipping**. If the vaporiser tips past 45° anaesthetic liquid can obstruct the valves and result in very high concentrations of vapour being delivered to the patient.
Solution	Take care when moving vaporisers. Regularly check the seating of the vaporiser on the back bar.

Describe the plenum vaporisers with electronic control.

These vaporisers are manufactured by GE, who have called them 'Aladin cassettes'. Although these cassettes look very different from the standard plenum vaporisers, they function in essentially the same manner and are colour-coded in the standard way. They can supply desflurane. Each cassette is a sump for anaesthetic liquid and the concentration of anaesthetic delivered to the patient depends on the splitting ratio of the free gas flowing through the cassette, just as in the 'ordinary' plenum vaporisers. Each different cassette plugs into a single slot in the front of the anaesthetic machine during use (i.e. one cassette is removed and replaced with another to change anaesthetic agent) and when it is inserted, it pushes open an inflow and an outflow valve.

The electronic control mechanism is situated inside the anaesthetic machine and the anaesthetist uses a digital display to programme the machine to deliver a specified concentration of anaesthetic or to target an end tidal concentration of anaesthetic agent.

These vaporisers are portable, can be tipped and are maintenance free but they cannot be used without power.

Why is it necessary to have a special vaporiser to deliver desflurane?

The physical properties of desflurane made it necessary to design its unique vaporiser. Desflurane is extremely volatile and its boiling point is 23 °C at atmospheric pressure, i.e. around room temperature. Because of its volatility, small changes in ambient temperature would result in large changes in desflurane's saturated vapour pressure (SVP) inside the vaporisation chamber and this would affect the concentration of anaesthetic agent delivered to the patient (*see* Chapter 62, 'States of matter' for a detailed explanation of this concept). This is not a problem with other volatile anaesthetic agents, because their boiling points are well above room temperature and so small variations in ambient temperature in theatre do not have a clinically significant effect on the SVP inside the vaporising chamber.

To overcome this problem, the desflurane vaporiser heats the anaesthetic agent to precisely 39 °C to ensure a constant SVP. Rather than free gas flowing into the vaporiser as in the plenum vaporisers, the anaesthetic vapour is injected into the free gas flow downstream of the vaporisation chamber. The anaesthetist will control the concentration of desflurane delivered to the patient using a dial calibrated from 0 to 12%. As the setting of the dial increases, the resistance to the flow of desflurane into the fresh gas flow decreases and more is injected, and vice versa. The rate of injection of desflurane must be adjusted according to the fresh gas flow otherwise turning the gas flow up would result in a dilution of the anaesthetic agent in the final gas mixture. This coupling is achieved by an electronic control unit in the vaporiser.

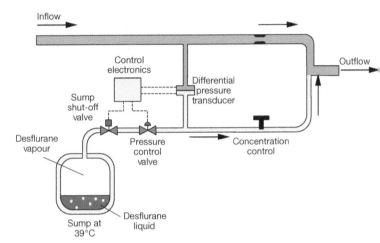

Fig. 77.3 Desflurane vaporiser

For completeness, we describe the DIVA (direct injection of volatile anaesthetic) vaporiser very briefly, although it's unlikely you'll be grilled about it...

The DIVA is a measured flow meter that can give all types of anaesthetic agent, including desflurane. In simple terms, the anaesthetic is heated to a specific temperature in an evaporation chamber before the vapour is passed into the patient gas circuit. As in the desflurane vaporiser, a microprocessor couples fresh gas flow to the rate of injection of the anaesthetic agent.

What considerations should be taken when building a vaporiser?

The properties of the anaesthetic to be delivered should be taken into account. These are explained above, but listed below:

- Saturated vapour pressure at room temperature
- Boiling point at atmospheric pressure
- MAC of anaesthetic agent: range on dial must increase with MAC such that:
  - Isoflurane   MAC = 1.15,   range 0–5%   on dial
  - Sevoflurane MAC = 2.10,   range 0–8%   on dial
  - Desflurane   MAC = 6.00,   range 0–12% on dial

How are vaporisers affected by altitude?

There is no clinical difference in using the plenum vaporiser at altitude, but the examiners seem to love this question because it brings out the physics in you! The answer below may be long-winded and obvious to many, but for the benefit of those of us who are mathematically challenged, here is the explanation in words of one syllable.

Please start by looking at chapter 62 for an explanation of SVP.

Plenum vaporisers (e.g. Tec 5 and 7)

Although we dial up the percentage of anaesthetic agent we want to deliver to the patient, it is not actually the percentage concentration of volatile being inhaled that determines whether a patient is anaesthetised, but the partial pressure of that volatile. Because we usually work at sea level at a pressure of 1 atmosphere, the values for 'percentage concentration' and 'partial pressure' delivered are happily inter-changeable (see proof below).

We can work out the partial pressure of a gas using Dalton's law of partial pressures, which states:

1 Each gas in a mixture exerts a pressure, known as its 'partial pressure', that is equal to the pressure the gas would exert if it were the only gas present. And for completeness, Dalton goes on to say:

2 The total pressure of the mixture is the sum of the partial pressures of all the gases present.

At sea level

So, the partial pressure of sevoflurane delivered as 4% of a gas mixture at sea level is:

- $P_{sevoflurane} = 4/100 \times 1$ atm $= 0.04$ atm (i.e. 4% of 1 atmosphere) and for completeness:
- $P_{total} = P_{sevoflurane} + P_{oxygen} + P_{nitrogen} + P_{other\ gases}$

The partial pressure of sevoflurane may also be expressed using different units of pressure, as follows:

- $P_{sevoflurane} = 4/100 \times 101.3$ kP$_a$ $= 4.05$ kP$_a$ (i.e. 4% of 101.3 kP$_a$)
- $P_{sevoflurane} = 4/100 \times 760$ torr $= 30.4$ torr (i.e. 4% of 760 torr)
- $P_{sevoflurane} = 4/100 \times 760$ mmHg $= 30.4$ mmHg (i.e. 4% of 760 mmHg)

Remembering that:

$$1 \text{ atm} = 101.3 \text{ kP}_a = 760 \text{ torr} = 760 \text{ mmHg}$$

Or:

$$0.04 \text{ atm} = 4.05 \text{ kP}_a = 30.4 \text{ torr} = 30.4 \text{ mmHg}$$

At altitude

At 5.5 km or 3.5 miles high, ambient partial pressure reduces to 0.5 atm.

If we take our vaporiser up to this altitude and set it again to deliver sevoflurane as 4% of the total gas mixture, we can use Dalton's law once more to work out the partial pressure of sevoflurane:

- $P_{sevoflurane} = 4/100 \times 0.5$ atm $= 0.02$ atm (i.e. 2% of 1 atmosphere)

We can see that the partial pressure of the sevoflurane has dropped by half. However, this is not the end of the story. At the top of our mountain, the ambient pressure of air has dropped by half. Since the pressure inside the vaporising chamber will be approximately equal to atmospheric pressure, as this falls, the concentration of the volatile agent delivered by the vaporiser will increase proportionately. The reasoning is described below, after a couple of facts have been emphasised:

1   SVP does **not** change with ambient pressure. It only changes with temperature.
2   The pressure inside the vaporising chamber will be approximately equal to the ambient air pressure (there must be a small difference in pressure between the two to cause flow of vapour out of the vaporiser).

Now consider the following three situations. In each, the only condition that changes is the altitude and consequently, the ambient air pressure. The temperature is kept at 20 °C. The SVP of sevoflurane at 20 °C is 100 mmHg (we will use mmHg in these calculations to make the numbers more manageable).

1   At sea level at 20 °C
  • Atmospheric pressure is 760 mmHg
  • SVP of sevoflurane is 100 mmHg

This means that, per unit volume of gas leaving the vaporising chamber, 100 'parts' of the 760 will be sevoflurane and 660 'parts' will be air.

This is true because Dalton's law states:

  • $P_{total} = P_{sevoflurane} + P_{air}$

and so

  • 760 mmHg = 100 mmHg + 660 mmHg

Therefore, the concentration of sevoflurane in the gas leaving the vaporiser is 100/750 = 13%.

2   At an altitude of 5.5 km at 20 °C
  • Atmospheric pressure is 380 mmHg
  • SVP of sevoflurane is 100 mmHg (unchanged)

This means that, per unit volume of gas leaving the vaporising chamber, 100 'parts' of the 380 will be sevoflurane and 280 'parts' will be air.

Therefore, the concentration of sevoflurane in the gas leaving the vaporiser is 100/380 = 26%.

3   At the bottom of a mine at 20 °C
  • Atmospheric pressure is say, 1000 mmHg
  • SVP of sevoflurane is 100 mmHg (unchanged)

This means that, per unit volume of gas leaving the vaporising chamber, 100 'parts' of the 1000 will be sevoflurane and 900 'parts' will be air.

Therefore, the concentration of sevoflurane in the gas leaving the vaporiser is 100/1000 = 10%.

So (finally!) we can see that a vaporiser calibrated at sea level and set to deliver 4% sevoflurane will actually deliver 8% at an altitude of 5.5 km. Since the partial pressure of 4% sevoflurane at 1 atmosphere/760 mmHg (0.04 atm/30.4 mmHg) is the same as 8% at 0.5 atmosphere/380 mmHg (0.04 atm/30.4 mmHg) the clinical effect of the sevoflurane on the patient remains the same. In this way, the anaesthetist can use the dial on the vaporiser in the usual way to achieve anaesthesia.

Simples…!?

The measured flow vaporiser (e.g. Tec 6) at 5.5 km altitude

Unfortunately, the same is not true of the Tec 6 vaporiser. As explained earlier, the Tec 6 heats desflurane to 39 °C to ensure that its SVP is constant and so fluctuations in ambient temperature do not result fluctuations in delivery of the anaesthetic agent. As a result, the SVP of desflurane inside this vaporising chamber at 39 °C is 2 atmospheres, regardless of ambient pressure.

Turning the dial on the Tec 6 vaporiser to 4% reflects the volume of gas that will be injected into the fresh gas flow to result in a gas mixture of 4% desflurane being delivered to the patient. However, as the desflurane leaves the vaporiser at altitude, this is 4% of a much lower ambient pressure and so the partial pressure of desflurane in the alveoli will be much lower.

Using Dalton's law again, we can see why this results in a drop in the partial pressure of desflurane being delivered when compared to sea level:

- $P_{desflurane} = 4/100 \times 0.5$ atm $= 0.02$ atm (i.e. 2% of 1 atmosphere)

Because of the way the vaporiser works, SVP remains constant at altitude. This means the anaesthetist will have to dial in a higher percentage of desflurane to achieve the same clinical effect at altitude as at sea level.

78. NEUROMUSCULAR BLOCKADE MONITORING

How can we assess the degree of neuromuscular blockade present in a patient?

It is important to know what degree of neuromuscular blockade is present in our patients so that we can manage the various stages of anaesthesia from tracheal intubation, muscle relaxation to facilitate safe surgery in the best possible conditions, the return of adequate spontaneous ventilation through to extubation.

Monitoring neuromuscular blockade involves two steps:

1 Stimulation of a motor nerve
2 Assessment of the muscular response

Stimulation of a motor nerve is be done clinically in two ways:

(i) Needle electrodes, e.g. Stimuplex needle, inserted into the tissue near the nerve. This method can be used to identify nerves to block during regional anaesthesia, although it is less commonly used now because ultrasound-guided regional anaesthesia has become popular. Here, the current applied to the nerve is low amplitude (1–3 mA to locate the general area of the nerve, reducing to 0.2–0.5 mA as the needle is brought nearer to the nerve prior to injection of local anaesthetic.)

(ii) Skin electrodes placed over a peripheral nerve, which deliver a supramaximal current (50 mA) to ensure recruitment of all muscle units.

After nerve stimulation, assessment of the resulting motor response is made. This assessment can be:

1 Visual/tactile: the anaesthetist observes 'twitches' and feels for muscle movement, e.g. holding the twitching thumb during ulnar nerve stimulation.
   - Advantages – simple, convenient, cheap
   - Disadvantages – prone to interpretation error, inaccurate, crude

2 Mechanomyography: a small weight is hung from the muscle to maintain isometric contraction. A strain gauge measures tension generated in the muscle following stimulation and converts it into an electrical signal. The tension generated is proportional to the force of contraction and so inversely proportional to the degree of neuromuscular blockade.
   - Advantages – more accurate than visual monitoring
   - Disadvantages – hand must be splinted and stable, fiddly and inconvenient. Used mainly in research

3 Acceleromyography: a transducer using piezoelectric crystals is secured to the end of a digit. The digit moves following stimulation and its acceleration is proportional to the force of muscle contraction and so inversely proportional to the degree of neuromuscular blockade.
- Advantages – more accurate than visual monitoring
- Disadvantages – hand must be splinted and stable, fiddly and inconvenient

4 Electromyography: a skin or needle electrode is placed over the adductor pollicis (this is the most commonly used muscle). The ulnar nerve is stimulated and the electrodes record the magnitude of the compound muscle action potentials generated as a consequence.
- Advantages – more accurate than visual monitoring. Avoids the problems of position and calibrating transducers attached to joints
- Disadvantages – even small movements of the hand can alter the response of the electrode

Tell me about the stimulation patterns used in neuromuscular monitoring.

It is easy to become confused by the seeming array of numbers and patterns that have to be learnt. In fact, this question is very simple, because all twitches that we deliver in theatre with the nerve stimulators are uniform and so you only have to learn a couple of facts.

- *All twitches are delivered at 50 mA (i.e. supramaximal stimulus)*
- *All twitches last 0.2 ms*

Once you have these facts, the rest becomes easier to remember.

In theatre, we mainly use visual and tactile assessment of the degree of neuromuscular blockade because of the relative convenience of this method. Several different patterns of stimulation have been developed to try to improve the sensitivity of monitoring. These are:

- Single twitch
- Train of four (TOF)
- Tetanic stimulation
- Post-tetanic count
- Double burst stimulation (DBS)

Single twitch

- Twitch current 50 mA
- Duration of twitch 0.2 ms
- Frequency of twitches 1 Hz (i.e. 1 every second)
- Number of twitches: as many as operator chooses to give

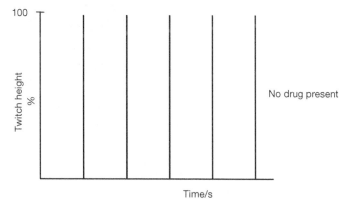

Fig. 78.1 Single twitch

This is the simplest stimulation pattern. At a frequency of 1 twitch per second, there is time for complete recovery of the muscle units between each stimulation. This means that we will not see 'fade' during single-twitch stimulation. Single twitch should be used before and after the administration of neuromuscular blocking drugs (NMBDs) to assess the degree of receptor occupancy by comparing the height of the twitch before drug administration and after. When 75% of the ACh receptors are occupied, the twice height starts to reduce; when 100% are occupied, there are no twitches at all.

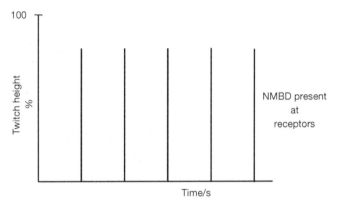

Fig. 78.2 Single twitch with competitive NMBD at receptor

Single twitch can be used to assess block in depolarising NMBD, i.e. suxamethonium, where fade and post-tetanic facilitation do not occur (*see* below).

Train of four (TOF)

- Twitch current 50 mA
- Duration of twitch 0.2 ms
- Frequency of twitches 2 Hz (i.e. 2 every second)
- Number of twitches: 4

In the TOF, the ratio of twitch height T4:T1 indicates the degree of receptor occupancy by the NMBD. Twitches height may be reduced or absent, and the disappearance of T4 = 75% occupancy, T3 = 80%, T2 + 90%, T1 = 100%. This phenomenon is called 'fade' (*see* below).

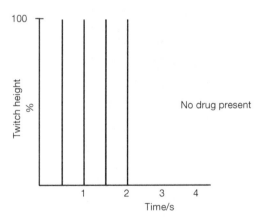

Fig. 78.3 Train of four

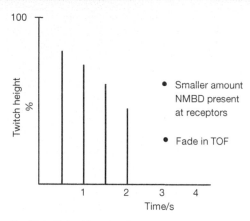

Fig. 78.4 Train of four – smaller amount of NMBD at receptor

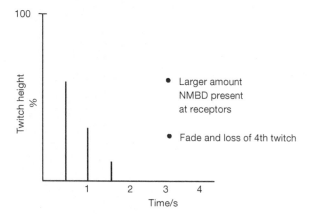

Fig. 78.5 Train of four – larger amount of NMBD at receptor

Accepted values for TOF:
- 1 twitch for tracheal intubation
- 1–2 twitches during surgery
- 3–4 twitches before attempting reversal with anticholinesterases

Tetanic stimulation
- Twitch current 50 mA
- Duration of twitch 0.2 ms
- Frequency of twitches 50 Hz (i.e. 50 every second)
- Number of twitches: stimulation lasts 5 seconds = $5 \times 50 = 250$ twitches

If neuromuscular block is present, tetanic stimulation will demonstrate fade inversely proportional to the percentage receptor occupation. Tetanic stimulation is applied before the tetanic count (*see* below). It is used to assess when there is profound block such that there are no twitches on TOF. Tetanic stimulation is extremely painful in an awake patient and may leave an unpleasant sensation in those who were anaesthetised.

Post-tetanic count (PTC)
- Twitch current 50 mA
- Duration of twitch 0.2 ms
- Frequency of twitches 1 Hz (i.e. 1 every second)
- Number of twitches: as many as operator chooses to give

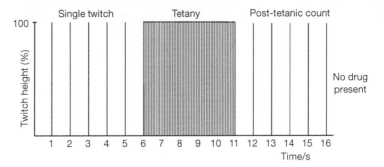

Fig. 78.6 Tetany – no NMBD present at receptor

The stimulation pattern here is identical to the single twitch. Following tetanic stimulation, post-tetanic facilitation mobilises presynaptic ACh, making it available to produce contractions in response to the current applied in the post-tetanic count (PTC). The number of twitches it is possible to produce is inversely proportional to the degree of receptor blockade.

- PTC <5 = profound block
- PTC >15 = equivalent to two twitches on TOF

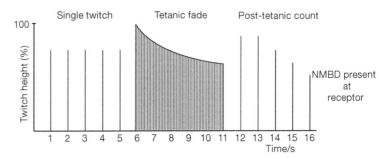

Fig. 78.7 Tetany – NMBD present at receptor

Double burst stimulation (DBS)

- Twitch current 50 mA
- Duration of twitch 0.2 ms
- Frequency of twitches 50 Hz (i.e. 50 every second)
- Number of twitches: 3 twitches – break of 750 ms – 3 more twitches

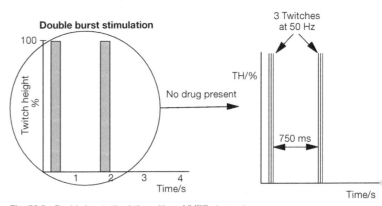

Fig. 78.8 Double burst stimulation with no NMBD at receptor

Double burst stimulation was developed to try to improve our ability to detect fade clinically, as the stimulation yields only two muscle contractions. It is easier for us to compare the heights of T1:T2 than detecting fade over four twitches.

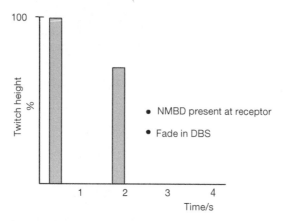

Fig. 78.9 Double burst stimulation with NMBD at receptor

What is fade?

'Fade' describes the phenomenon of decreasing twitch height when competitive neuromuscular blocking drugs are present at the neuromuscular junction (NMJ).

ACh is stored in vesicles in the terminal button at the NMJ. Each vesicle contains over 10 000 ACh molecules. Eighty per cent of the vesicles are readily releasable, while 20% form a stationary store. At the normal NMJ, the arrival of an action potential of sufficient magnitude will cause >100 vesicles to fuse with the pre-synaptic membrane and discharge their ACh into the synaptic cleft. The ACh diffuses across the cleft, binds to post-synaptic ACh receptors and triggers the muscle AP, which causes contraction. In addition to the post-synaptic ACh receptors, there are pre-junctional receptors found on the terminal button. These too are stimulated by the release of ACh and, in the face of repeated APs, they have a positive feedback role by stimulating an increase in ACh production by second messenger systems. This helps to prevent the muscle fatigue with prolonged stimulation.

When molecules of NMBD are bound to the post-synaptic ACh receptors, it leaves fewer for the ACh to bind to. There is a large safely margin at the NMJ and there will be no discernible weakness until 75% of receptor sites are occupied. Fade occurs when there is sufficient NMBD present to compete significantly with binding of ACh at both the pre and post-synaptic receptors. Binding of the drug to the pre-synaptic receptors prevents the positive feedback mechanism, which results in increased production of ACh. Consequently, a decreasing amount of ACh is released with each stimulation and this is reflected in a decreasing twitch height: so called 'fade'.

What is post-tetanic potentiation?

Tetanic stimulation is a supra-maximal stimulation, applied to the NMJ for a prolonged period of time. It is sufficient to produce a substantial increase in ACh release, enough to overcome competition from NMBD in all but the most profound of blocks. The positive feedback mechanism described above is activated and this increases the amount of ACh available for release. This is called post-tetanic potentiation.

What are phase I and phase II blocks?	These terms refer to the blocks seen following the administration of suxamethonium.

A phase I block describes the block seen following the administration of a single dose of suxamethonium. Suxamethonium binds to the ACh receptor, which causes opening of the sodium channel and membrane depolarisation. This results in disorganised muscle contraction, seen as fasciculation followed by flaccid paralysis because suxamethonium causes prolonged depolarisation of the motor end plate.

The characteristics of a phase I block:

- Reduced twitch height, but sustained response to tetanic stimulation
- No post-tetanic facilitation
- TOF ratio >70% (height of fourth twitch to that of first). This is a measure of the pre-synaptic effect of suxamethonium.

The block is potentiated by the effect of anticholinesterases because these will further decrease the rate of suxamethonium breakdown.

A phase II block describes the block seen following the repeated administration/infusion of suxamethonium and can develop with doses in excess of 2.5 mg/kg. It occurs because in the continued presence of suxamethonium, the receptors eventually close and the membrane repolarises, at least partially. However, it is now desensitised to ACh and so cannot open again to propagate an action potentials. In this way, a phase II block is similar to a non-depolarising block. Phase II blocks are also called 'desensitisation blocks'.

Characteristics of a phase II block:

- Exhibits fade on tetanic stimulation
- Exhibits post-tetanic facilitation
- TOF ratio <0.3 (fourth to first twitch height)
- Antagonised by anticholinesterases
- Tachyphylaxis is seen with the need to increase suxamethonium infusion rate or bolus dose.

Which nerves can we monitor clinically?

Commonly monitored nerves in theatre are:

- Facial nerve – twitch of the eyebrow with orbicularis oculi contraction
- Ulnar nerve – twitch of the thumb with adductor pollicis contraction
- Posterior tibial nerve – twitch of the big toe with flexor hallucis brevis contraction.

Which muscles are affected first by NMBDs?

NMBDs cause paralysis of all voluntary muscles in the body, but some are more sensitive than others. In order of decreasing sensitivity:

- Eyes (affected first)
- Facial muscles
- Neck
- Extremities
- Limbs
- Abdominal muscles
- Glottis
- Intercostal muscles (affected last).

Muscle function returns in the reverse order. This is why it is traditional to wait until a patient can lift their head of the pillow before extubation.

79. LASERS

What do you understand by the term 'laser'?	Laser is an acronym for 'light amplification by the stimulated emission of radiation'. Lasers produce an intense beam of light that is monochromatic (single wavelength), coherent (in phase) and collimated (parallel). Laser technology allows high-energy intensities to be produced from relatively low-power sources.
Describe the basic physics underpinning laser technology.	> The quantum theory states that electrons are confined to certain energy states but these electrons can move between these energy states depending on whether they absorb or emit energy. > Einstein demonstrated that if you stimulated an atom with a photon of energy, this stimulated atom would in turn emit a photon of equivalent energy, which was in phase with the original stimulating photon. This new emitted photon could now cause a further similar reaction and as such a chain reaction and hence amplification of the system would ensue. > In lasers, an external source of energy (e.g. high voltage or flash of light) is applied to a laser medium. > This increases the energy state of the electrons within the laser medium and moves them up from a 'ground' energy state to an 'excited' energy state. > When these excited electrons return to their original ground state they emit energy in the form of light or radiation. > This emitted energy can then stimulate further electrons within the medium, thereby amplifying the whole process. > The wavelength of light produced depends on the lasing medium that is used.
What are the fundamental components within a laser device?	> External energy source (to 'stimulate' the electrons) > Laser medium (this can be a solid, liquid or a gas) > Chamber containing the laser medium > System of mirrors (to allow 'amplification' of radiation) > A partially reflective mirror (to allow the emitted radiation to exit the system) > Windows at each end of the device are inclined to Brewster's angle (this is the angle of incidence at which light is perfectly transmitted with no reflection, thereby ensuring that 100% of the light is transmitted through the windows) > Fibre-optic cable (to direct the laser beam).
List the different types of lasers with their clinical applications.	> **Nd-YAG (neodymium-doped-yttrium aluminium garnet) lasers** • Crystal used as a lasing medium in solid-state lasers. • Wavelength of light produced is 1064 nm (near infrared region). • Good tissue penetration (as it is not absorbed by water). • Used typically for endoscopic surgery (there have been reports of inadvertent pneumothoraces during ENT surgery due to these lasers penetrating and affecting tissues deeper than anticipated).

> **Carbon dioxide lasers**
>   - Used as a lasing medium in gas-state lasers.
>   - Highest power laser currently available (also used in industry for cutting, welding and engraving).
>   - Wavelength of light produced is 10.6 μm (infrared region).
>   - Poor tissue penetration of <200 μm (as it is absorbed by water causing it to vaporise and destroy tissue contents).
>   - Used typically for superficial surgery (e.g. dermabrasion and laser 'facelifts').
>   - Unsuitable for endoscopic use.

> **Argon lasers**
>   - Used as a lasing medium in gas-state lasers.
>   - Wavelength of light produced is between 400 and 700 nm (blue-green region of the visible spectrum).
>   - Good penetration through transparent tissues (e.g. aqueous humour, vitreous humour and lens of the eye).
>   - Maximally absorbed by red-pigmented tissues (e.g. birthmarks, haemoglobin).
>   - Used typically in eye surgery (e.g. retinal phototherapy) and in dermatological procedures to cosmetically enhance pigmented lesions.

> **Dye lasers**
>   - Organic dye used as a lasing medium in liquid-state lasers.
>   - Wavelength of light produced is broad and varies occurring to the dye used.
>   - Used typically in 'beauty clinics' to even out skin tone.

How are lasers classified?

> **Class 1** – power does not exceed maximum permissible exposure for the eye.
> **Class 2** – power up to 1 mW and visible laser beams only. Eye protected by blink reflex.
> **Class 3a** – power up to 5 mW and visible spectrum only but now laser beam must be expanded (so that maximum irradiance does not exceed 25 W/m^2); eyes protected by blink reflex.
> **Class 3b** – power up to 0.5 W and any wavelength; direct viewing hazardous; dye protection essential.
> **Class 4** – power > 0.5 W and any wavelength; extremely hazardous and capable of igniting inflammable materials; eye protection essential.

What are the hazards of laser surgery?

Lasers are hazardous to use because they combine high-energy intensities confined within a small spot size (i.e. very concentrated) and transmitted in a non-divergent beam (i.e. these devices do not lose power with increasing distance from the laser source). For comparison, when looking directly into sunlight the eye is exposed to approximately 150 W/m^2 but if inadvertently looking into a laser beam, the eye is exposed to approximately 3×10^6 W/m^2!

> **Environment:**
>   - Fire and explosions – flammable spirits, oxygen and nitrous oxide can get collected in the drapes and these can get ignited if the laser beam is directed to it.

> **Staff:**
>   - Eyes – if the laser beam hits the retina, a permanent blind spot can develop, but if it hits the optic nerve permanent blindness can be caused (CO_2 lasers do not penetrate the cornea and therefore cannot affect the retina).
>   - Skin – if the laser beam hits the skin, a burning sensation is felt and this will trigger self-protecting manoeuvres.

> **Laser hazards affecting the anaesthetised patient:**
> * Eyes – as above.
> * Skin – now self-protecting manoeuvres do not come to play and therefore patients are at risk of laser burns.
> * Airway fire – this is a real risk during laser surgery to the upper airway (this is an anaesthetic emergency and therefore you must be well versed with both the precautions needed to prevent this and the immediate management required to deal with this).

What precautions are taken to minimise the hazards of laser surgery?

> **General:**
> * Designated laser protection supervisor for each theatre
> * Staff all trained and educated in laser use
> * Doors locked, windows closed and signs displayed to protect those outside theatre.

> **Equipment:**
> * Eye protection goggles (laser beam wavelength-specific) for both staff and patient
> * Surgical instruments with a black or matt finish to minimise refection of laser beam.

> **Anaesthetic considerations for upper airway laser surgery:**
> * Double-cuffed, laser-resistant endotracheal tube (these are often flexible stainless steel tubes with two cuffs to ensure a tracheal seal if the upper cuff is accidentally damaged by the laser)
> * Cuffs filled with saline (air-filled cuffs may ignite if hit by the laser)
> * Throat packed with wet swabs (to protect adjacent areas from inadvertent laser burns)
> * Oxygen – air mix (as nitrous oxide is more flammable)
> * $FiO_2 < 0.25$ if tolerated

What are the basic concepts in managing an airway fire?

> Call for help and inform your immediate theatre team.
> Surgeon to switch off laser and flood the operation site with water.
> Disconnect the anaesthetic machine.
> Remove endotracheal tube if feasible (remember that even laser-resistant tubes can ignite).
> Ventilate the patient with a bag-valve-mask circuit (if necessary continue anaesthesia with TIVA).
> Surgeon to inspect the airway with rigid bronchoscope.
> Refer to ITU (airway fires can cause significant lung injury and ARDS – patient may require ventilation, dexamethasone, and humidified oxygen).

80. ULTRASOUND AND DOPPLER

What are the clinical uses of ultrasound?

In the last decade there has been a rapid expansion in the use of ultrasound within anaesthetics and critical care medicine. Use of ultrasound has become routine in the theatre environment to aid vascular line insertion (NICE 2002), guide peripheral nerve blockade, e.g. interscalene nerve blocks (NICE 2009), and in some centres to also guide catheter placement within the epidural space (NICE 2008). In the critical care setting, ultrasound is routinely used for vascular line insertion, cardiac output monitoring, echocardiography, transcranial Doppler, pleural aspiration, ascitic drainage, assessment of hepatic portal vein flow and detection of venous thromboembolism.

What are the principles of ultrasound?

> Ultrasound is an imaging modality that utilises high-frequency sound waves (in the region of 2 MHz) in order to image structures within the body.
> Ultrasound waves are generated by applying an electric field to a piezoelectric crystal in the transducer, which leads to the crystal vibrating and generating ultrasound waves.
> Tissues within the body differ in their ability to transmit sound waves. When the sound wave encounters a change in tissue, part of the sound wave is transmitted and part is reflected back to the transducer. It is the reflected sound waves that are converted into an image. The time taken for the sound waves to return to the transducer provides an indication of the depth of the tissue, interface.
> Ultrasound gel is essential to acquire good images, acting as a coupling medium, which reduces the attenuation of the ultrasound waveform.
> Ultrasound is good for examining fluid-filled structures (e.g. vessels) and soft tissues, but not for air-filled structures (e.g. lung tissue) or for calcium-rich structures (e.g. bone).
> Resolution of the ultrasound image is inversely proportional to the depth of penetration and so it is not good for examining deep structures or imaging obese patients.
> Advantages: relatively inexpensive, widely available, non-invasive and no ionising radiation, therefore safe in children and pregnancy.
> Disadvantages: operator dependent, cannot be used to image lung, bone or deep structures.

What are the different modes of ultrasound?	Several different modes of ultrasound are utilised in medical imaging, the main ones are described below:

> **A (Amplitude) Mode** – simplest form of ultrasound imaging that is not frequently used. A single ultrasound wave is emitted from the probe and scans a line through the body with the echoes plotted on the screen as a function of depth. Used by ophthalmologists to measure diameter of the eyeball.

> **B (Brightness) Mode** (better known as 2D mode) – a linear array of ultrasound waves are emitted from the probe and scan a section through the body producing a two-dimensional cross-sectional view. The intensity of the echoes reflected back to the transducer is proportional to the whitening of the film, thus structures with no internal echoes appear black (anechoic) whereas structures containing internal echoes appear white (echogenic). It is the default mode of any ultrasound or echocardiography machine. This mode is used widely in anaesthetic practice to gain vascular access and to perform regional anaesthesia. In echocardiography, it is used to measure cardiac chambers and to visualise valves.

> **M (Motion) Mode** – a rapid sequence of ultrasound waves are emitted and each time either an A-mode or B-mode image is taken allowing real-time movement of structures to be visualised. This mode is commonly used in echocardiography.

> **Doppler Mode** – utilises the Doppler effect to enable detection and velocity of flow. Sound waves reflected from a moving target (e.g. blood) have a different frequency from the incident sound wave. This frequency shift is proportional to the velocity of the flowing blood. Doppler allows not only the detection of flowing blood but also enables its velocity to be quantified.

- Colour flow Doppler – in this mode the velocity and direction of blood flow is colour coded and superimposed onto a grey-scale 2-D (B-mode) image. By convention **B**lue indicates flow '**A**way' from the ultrasound probe and **R**ed '**T**owards' the probe (acronym 'BART').
- Duplex Doppler – this mode combines real-time Doppler with real-time ultrasound simultaneously. Most commonly used to assess the vasculature (e.g. carotid occlusive disease, deep vein thrombosis, varicose veins, abdominal aortic aneurysms).

Define the Doppler effect.	Doppler effect (or principle) is a commonly observed phenomenon whereby sound waves reflected from a moving target are altered and have a different frequency from the incident sound wave. A good example of this is the noise of a racing car where the pitch (frequency) of the car increases as it approaches the observer and then abruptly drops as it races past the observer (but to the driver, the pitch will remain unchanged).
Give an equation to describe the Doppler effect.	In clinical ultrasonography, if the ultrasound beam is directed parallel to the direction of movement or flow, the velocity of the moving target (e.g. blood) is calculated as follows:

$$\text{Velocity} = \frac{\text{Speed of sound wave} \times \text{(change in frequency)}}{\text{(2} \times \text{emitted frequency)}}$$

Or:

$$V = c\,(\Delta f)/2f$$

Where:
c = speed of sound wave
f = frequency

> When the beam cannot be parallel to the direction of flow, a correction factor is used that involves the cosine of the angle of incidence (represented as θ). So now it is expressed as:

$$V = c(\Delta f)/2f \cos \theta$$

Give a clinical example of a
device utilising ultrasound.

> **Transoesophageal Doppler**
- This has now become established as a relatively non-invasive method of cardiac output monitoring.
- Doppler probe is positioned in the mid-oesophagus in order to measure red blood cell velocity in the descending thoracic aorta.
- Aortic cross-sectional area is estimated from a nomogram (age/height/weight) or in some devices it is measured.
- Once the probe is positioned correctly, it uses the Doppler principle to measure red blood cell velocity from which blood flow can then be calculated.

81. CT AND MRI

A transfer to the CT or MRI scanner with an anaesthetised patient is not a task to be undertaken lightly. There is good reason why the CT scanner is sometimes referred to as the 'doughnut of death'. When answering a question on scan transfers, it is important to show the examiners that you are well prepared to cope with the potential pitfalls that may occur on your journey.

What are the principles behind computed tomography (CT) scanning?

The name comes from the Greek 'tomo', meaning slice and 'graphein', to write. CTs take a series of X-ray images around a central axis, either in a discontinuous 'shoot and step' process, or in a continuous 'spiral' manner. The latter are much quicker and so may reduce motion artefact, and enable better 3D reconstruction of images.

What are the principles behind magnetic resonance imaging (MRI)?

> MRI is an alternative way of producing images of the body.
> MRI visualises soft tissues much better than does CT, and therefore is more useful in the study of the brain, spinal cord and musculoskeletal system.
> Atoms with unpaired electrons or protons are in a state of spin that can be affected by the application of an external magnetic field.
> Hydrogen ions found in water and fat molecules (which make up 60–70% of the body) are affected in this way and so, when the patient enters the powerful magnetic field of the scanner (1–2 tesla), their protons align in the direction of the field.
> The protons then begin to resonate at their 'precision frequency'.
> The powerful magnet is called the 'primary magnet' and its magnetic field is generated by an electrical current passing through coils of wire, which are cooled with liquid helium.
> Once the atoms have lined up, a radiofrequency coil is turned on, generating a second current at right angles to the first.
> The energy generated by this coil is absorbed by the hydrogen ions and disrupts their alignment.
> When the radiofrequency coil is turned off, the protons release energy (in the form of low-frequency radiation) and return to their original position.
> It is this low-frequency radiation that is detected by the scanner, and reconstructed into images.
> Different tissues will give out different amounts of energy and return to their equilibrium position at different rates, allowing for differentiation between them. This exchange of energy between spin states is called 'resonance'.
> Another component of the MRI scanner is the 'gradient magnet'. These are smaller magnets that are applied to allow fine-tuning and focusing of the image on the area being studied. The banging noise in the MRI is the sound of these magnets being turned on and off.

> MRIs are either T1 or T2 weighted and this refers to the amount of time elapsed between the radiofrequency magnet being switched off and the image being taken, i.e. the 'relaxation time'. T1 images are taken earlier than T2. In T1 images fat is bright and water is black, in T2 images fat is black and water is bright.

> The entire scanner is housed in a room lined with copper or aluminium, and this room is referred to as the Faraday cage.

> What are the indications for general anaesthesia in the scanner?

> Unstable patient (e.g. for airway protection or from ITU)

> Young child if they cannot cooperate and lie still

> Patient with learning difficulties, as above

> Very anxious or claustrophobic patient

> Patients with movement disorders or who are unable to lie still for sufficiently long.

What are the problems associated with anaesthesia in the scanning department?

> Generic problems:

- **Patients are removed to an often remote and isolated area:** This area may be unfamiliar to the responsible doctor. It is important, therefore, to consider who will be available to help should there be an emergency during the trip and if possible, to familiarise oneself with the department and the equipment available there before the transfer.

- **Cold and noisy environment:** Ambient temperature in an MRI scanner is cool in order to prevent the magnet from overheating. The magnets produce a lot of noise and earplugs must therefore be used and patients covered in order to minimise risk of hypothermia.

- **Claustrophobic environment:** Space within scanners is extremely limited, more so in the MRI scanner, and some patients can find this very distressing.

- **Limited space for anaesthetic equipment**

- **Limited access to the patient:** Once the patient is in the scanner it can be practically impossible to get to them. Before the scan begins it is important to satisfy yourself that all the leads reach far enough, that the patient is stable and that you can see the monitor. The scan may take some time, especially if it is an MRI.

> **Specific problems related to the MRI scanner:** The magnet in the MRI adds a whole new layer of problems.

- **Ferrous implants:** Within the magnetic field, ferrous implants (e.g. pacemakers, defibrillators, cochlear implants, some aneurysm clips and foreign bodies) are prone to displacement or torque forces, which can lead to serious patient injury. Patients with any such implants must not enter the MRI scanner. Non-ferrous implants are prone to heating and patients must be warned of this. Both types of implants can cause image artefacts.

- **Ferrous equipment:** Ferrous-containing equipment such as laryngoscopes, stethoscopes, pagers, and gas cylinders are prone to significant movement within the 50 G line and should therefore not be taken beyond this point unless securely fastened. Magnetic strips on identity badges and credit cards will also be wiped if taken within the magnetic field. Ideally, only 'MR safe' and 'MR conditional' equipment should be used within the scanner.

- **Monitoring:** Special 'MR safe' ECG electrodes, BP cuffs and pulse oximeters are required. ECG leads are short and plaited to minimise the risk of magnetically induced currents within them, which can burn the patient (burns are the most common MRI-associated injury). If a standard anaesthetic machine is used, this is housed outside the Faraday cage with an extra long Bain circuit connecting it to the patient. Long gas analysis sampling lines cause a delay in monitoring. Monitoring equipment can introduce stray radiofrequency currents, which can degrade the image quality.

- **Delivery of anaesthesia:** 'MR conditional' infusion pumps should ideally be used. However, standard pumps can also be used outside the 100 G line (*see* below). Volatile agents can be administered using an 'MR conditional' anaesthetic machine. If this is not available, a standard anaesthetic machine can be used outside the cage with an extra-long Bain circuit.

How are items to be used within an MRI scanner classified?

The old term 'MR compatible' is no longer suitable and the ASTM International and FDA have introduced the following classification system:

> **MR Safe:** Items are completely free of all metallic components. They are non-metallic, non-conductive and non-radiofrequency reactive. They pose no hazard in any MR environment.

> **MR Conditional:** Items are safe under certain tested magnetic conditions, which should be enumerated on the product (i.e. the magnetic field strength in which the product can be safely used is stated).

> **MR Unsafe:** Items pose a hazard in any MR environment.

What is the standard international unit of magnetic strength?

> SI unit for magnetic flux is the weber (Wb)

> SI unit for magnetic flux density is the tesla (T), which is used for large densities. For smaller densities, a smaller unit, the gauss (G) is used. An average MR scanner produces between 1 and 1.5 T (although newer machines can now generate up to 3–5 T), while earth's magnetic field is about 1 G.

$$1\ T = 1\ Wb/m^2$$
$$1\ T = 10\ 000\ gauss$$

82. PULSE OXIMETRY

What is a pulse of oximeter and how does it work?

A pulse oximeter is a piece of equipment used to measure the percentage of arterial haemoglobin in the blood, which is saturated with oxygen (HbO_2 sats).

The equipment consists of an electronic processor, two light-emitting diodes (LEDs) and a photodiode. The LEDs and the photodiode are usually arranged on either end of an adhesive strip, or on a 'clip', that is placed around a thin part of the patient's anatomy, typically a finger, an ear lobe or the forefoot of an infant. The light from the LEDs shines through the patient and is detected by the photodiode.

Each LED emits light at a different frequency: one at 660 nm (red light) and the other at 940 nm (infrared light). Oxyhaemoglobin and deoxyhaemoglobin absorb these wavelengths of light differently; this is why arterial blood appears brighter red than venous blood to the human eye.

- Oxyhaemoglobin absorbs more infrared light (940 nm) and allows more red light (660 nm) to pass through.
- Deoxyhaemoglobin absorbs more red light (660 nm) and allows more infrared light (940 nm) to pass through.

The LEDs flash in sequence: one on, then the other, then both off to allow correction for ambient light. This triplet sequence happens 30 times per second. The amount of light transmitted through the patient at each frequency is detected by the photodiode. The microprocessor corrects for ambient light, and also for the difference between arterial and venous saturations by deducting the minimum transmitted light, during diastole, from the maximum during systole.

After this, the ratio of oxy- to deoxyhaemoglobin is determined and from this the percentage oxygen saturations using an empirically determined table derived from healthy volunteers who were exposed to varying degrees of hypoxia.

Whose law is used in this calculation?

Beer-Lambert law, which relates the attenuation of light to the properties of the material through which the light is travelling. It is used to calculate the absorbance of a solution.

The law states that the absorbance of a solution depends on:

- The concentration of that solution, i.e. the more molecules of a light-absorbing compound there are in the sample, the more light will be absorbed.
- The path-length of light travelling through the solution, i.e. the longer the length of the sample container, the more light will be absorbed because the light will come into contact with more molecules.

This is most simply expressed below:

$$A = \varepsilon lc$$

Where **A** is absorbance of the solution and $A = \log_{10} I_0/I$. I is the light intensity of the wavelength being passed through the solution. If I is less than I_0, then a proportion of the original light must have been absorbed by the solution.

ε is the molar absorption coefficient (L mol^{-1} cm^{-1}). It compensates for variance in concentration and the path-length to allow comparison between solutions.

I is the length of solution that the light passes through.

c is the concentration of the compound in solution, expressed in mol L^{-1}

Can you draw a graph comparing the absorbance of light by oxyhaemoglobin with deoxyhaemoglobin?

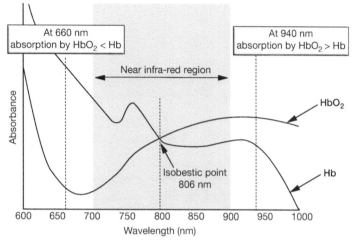

Fig. 82.1 Absorption spectra of oxy and deoxyhaemoglobin for red and infrared light

What factors may decrease the accuracy of pulse oximetry?

The following may cause erroneously low readings:

- Poor perfusion: hypotension/vasoconstriction
- Movement artefact
- Electrical interference from diathermy
- Highly calloused skin
- Nail varnish/artificial nails
- Severe anaemia
- Cardiac arrhythmias
- Methaemoglobinaemia – characteristically cause saturations to be measured at around 85%
- Increased venous pulsation, e.g. severe tricuspid regurgitation
- Intravenous administration of methylene blue dye because it absorbs light in the 660–670 nm range.

The following may cause high readings:

- Carbon monoxide poisoning – CO irreversibly binds to haemoglobin
- Cyanide poisoning – this is not inaccurate. Cyanide prevents oxygen being utilised in respiration and so its extraction from the blood falls, meaning saturations are high.

Miscellaneous factors:

- The human volunteers used to construct empirical saturation tables did not have their oxygen saturations dropped below approximately 85%; hence readings below this number are extrapolated, not validated.

Of note, fetal haemoglobin and HbS (sickle) do not affect readings.

INDEX